APhA's Immunization Handbook

3rd Edition

American Pharmacists Association Books and Electronic Products

Mission Statement

Our mission is to provide engaging resources for the profession to advance patient care and improve medication use.

We will achieve this by

- Providing the profession with authoritative content
- Offering products that enhance patient care, practice management, and leadership in the profession
- Delivering innovative solutions for the market
- Serving our members with the tools needed for continuing professional development

Disclaimer/Notices

The author and the publisher have made every effort to ensure the accuracy and completeness of the information presented in this book. However, the author and the publisher cannot be held responsible for the continued currency of the information or the application of this information, nor can they ensure that every vaccine available for distribution in the United States is discussed herein. Readers are encouraged to consult current recommendations of the Centers for Disease Control and Prevention and the Advisory Committee on Immunization Practices, as well as vaccine product package inserts.

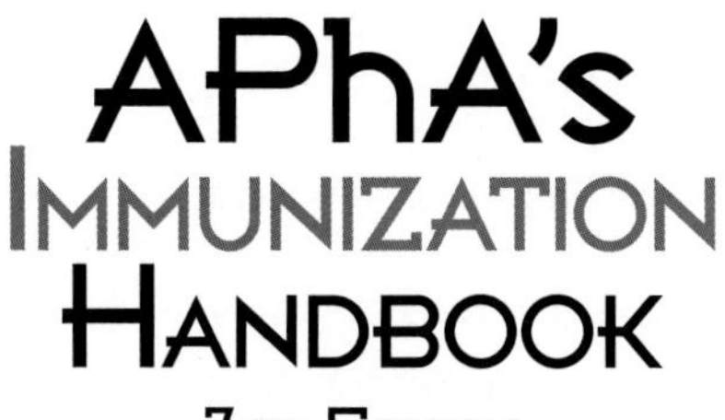

APhA's Immunization Handbook

3rd Edition

Lauren B. Angelo, PharmD, MBA

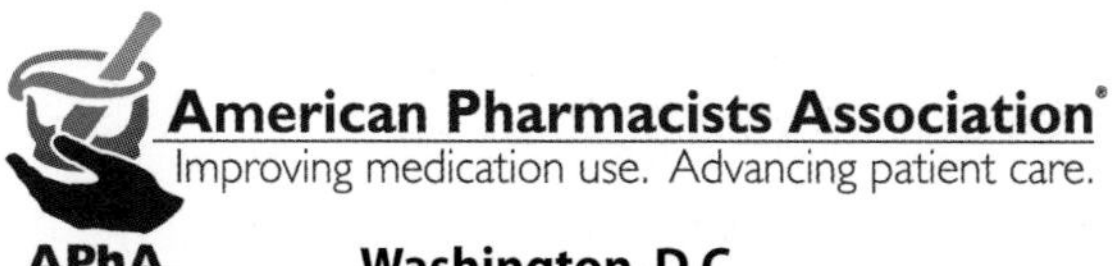

Washington, D.C.

Editor: Nancy Tarleton Landis
Acquiring Editor: Julian I. Graubart
Cover Design: Scott Neitzke, APhA Integrated Design and Production Center
Composition: Circle Graphics
Proofreading: Kathleen K. Wolter
Indexing: Suzanne Peake

APhA was founded in 1852 as the American Pharmaceutical Association.

Published by the American Pharmacists Association, 2215 Constitution Avenue, NW, Washington, DC 20037-2985

www.pharmacist.com www.pharmacylibrary.com

To comment on this book via e-mail, send your message to the publisher at aphabooks@aphanet.org.

Library of Congress Cataloging-in-Publication Data
Angelo, Lauren B., author.
APhA's immunization handbook / Lauren B. Angelo. — 3rd edition.
p. ; cm.
American Pharmacists Association's immunization handbook
Includes bibliographical references and index.
ISBN 978-1-58212-242-7
I. American Pharmacists Association, issuing body. II. Title. III. Title: American Pharmacists Association's immunization handbook.
[DNLM: 1. Immunization Programs--organization & administration—United States—Handbooks. 2. Pharmaceutical Services—organization & administration—United States—Handbooks. 3. Immunization—methods—United States—Handbooks. QV 735]
RA638
614.4'70973—dc23
2015001627

How to Order This Book

Online: www.pharmacist.com/shop
By phone: 800-878-0729 (770-280-0085 from outside the United States)
VISA®, MasterCard®, and American Express® cards accepted

Contents

Guide to Tables and Figures

Preface

Since the 2012 publication of this handbook's second edition, a great deal of attention and resources have been devoted to increasing immunization rates. We are now several years closer to 2020 and the Healthy People 2020 goals.[1] We have made progress over the past few years, but we are not quite there.

The 2012 data for adults—the patient population most pharmacists are likely to be vaccinating—show that vaccination rates are alarmingly low. They are so low, in fact, that I had to read those findings twice to make sure I was interpreting them correctly. Pneumococcal vaccination in high-risk adults age 19–64 was 20%; in patients 65 and older it was 60%. The Healthy People 2020 goals are 60% and 90%, respectively. Herpes zoster vaccination for those age 60 and older seems most likely to be on target at 20%, given that the goal is only 30%. The data for childhood and adolescent vaccination appear more encouraging. The one area that lags considerably behind, however, is human papillomavirus vaccination in adolescents. The goal for females age 13–15 is 80% for all three doses of the vaccine, but the rate for those age 15 was only 40%.[2] Granted, guidelines and recommendations have changed over the years and it may take some time to catch up, but the available data are rather concerning.

Although the 2020 goal for influenza vaccination of pregnant women has not been set, it is interesting to note that half of women who were pregnant during the 2012–2013 influenza season went unvaccinated.[3] In a survey of the pregnant women who received the vaccine, 71% reported receiving both a provider recommendation to be vaccinated and an offer of vaccine administration. Of the women given a recommendation to receive the vaccine but not an offer of vaccine administration, only 46% were vaccinated. Providers' ability to not only recommend vaccine to these women but also administer it seems to have had a profound impact.

As health care providers, we have a gap to close in our own vaccination rates. The Healthy People 2020 influenza vaccination goal for health care personnel (HCP) is 90%. During the 2012–2013 influenza season, only 72% of HCP received the influenza vaccine.[4] The vaccination rate was 89% for pharmacists, 85% for nurses, and 92% for physicians—not far from the 2020 goal. Other clinical and nonclinical personnel had lower rates, however. These individuals may not be administering vaccines, but they work in health care facilities and interact with patients on a regular basis, and thus they are included in the analysis. They are our employees, co-workers, and team members. As immunizing pharmacists, we should encourage them to be vaccinated. The overall HCP vaccination rate has increased over the years, and our support and advocacy will help continue this upward trend.

The Immunization Action Coalition (IAC) has a Web page listing evidence-based resources for assessing and improving immunization rates, at www.immunize.org/journalarticles/serv_ass.asp. IAC has also created a page specifically for pharmacists, at www.immunize.org/pharmacists. The Centers for Disease Control and Prevention (CDC) also offers sites and resources to help providers increase immunization rates, with an enhanced focus on the use of reminder, recall, and immunization information systems. Two examples are Reminder Systems and Strategies for Increasing Childhood Vaccination Rates, available at www.cdc.gov/vaccines/recs/reminder-sys.htm, and Strategies for Increasing Adult Vaccination Rates, available at www.cdc.gov/vaccines/hcp/patient-ed/adults/for-practice/increasing-vacc-rates.html. Promotional tools and resources such as these are referred to throughout this book to remind pharmacists of the important role we play as immunization advocates.

Every chapter in this edition of the handbook has been updated, and major changes and additions include the following:

- Greater focus on increasing immunization rates
- Reorganization of chapters to enhance the conceptual flow of content
- A new chapter dedicated to recommendations for immunocompromised and high-risk patients
- Updated Web links and sites
- Revised storage, handling, and administration guidance
- Modified billing information, codes, and resources
- Additional sources of primary literature to support pharmacists' efforts to increase vaccination rates

- New questions and answers from the IAC's "Ask the Experts" forum
- Updated vaccine product information
- New vaccination schedules

This third edition of *APhA's Immunization Handbook* would not have been possible without the encouragement, perspectives, and suggestions I have received from reviewers and avid users of the book. Please keep providing your comments—both positive and constructive. They are greatly appreciated and will be taken into account for the next edition.

References

1. U.S. Department of Health and Human Services. Healthy People 2020 Topics & Objectives: Immunization and Infectious Diseases. www.healthypeople.gov/2020/topics-objectives/topic/immunization-and-infectious-diseases/objectives. Accessed October 16, 2014.

2. Centers for Disease Control and Prevention. National, regional, state, and selected local area vaccination coverage among adolescents aged 13–17 years—United States, 2013. *MMWR Morb Mortal Wkly Rep.* 2014;63(29):625–33.

3. Centers for Disease Control and Prevention. Influenza vaccination coverage among pregnant women—United States, 2012–2013 influenza season. *MMWR Morb Mortal Wkly Rep.* 2013;62(38):787–92.

4. Centers for Disease Control and Prevention. Influenza vaccination coverage among health-care personnel—United States, 2012–2013 influenza season. *MMWR Morb Mortal Wkly Rep.* 2013;62(38):781–6.

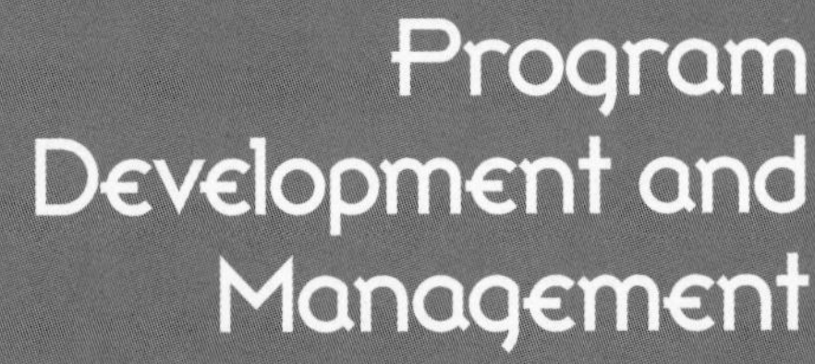

Program Development and Management

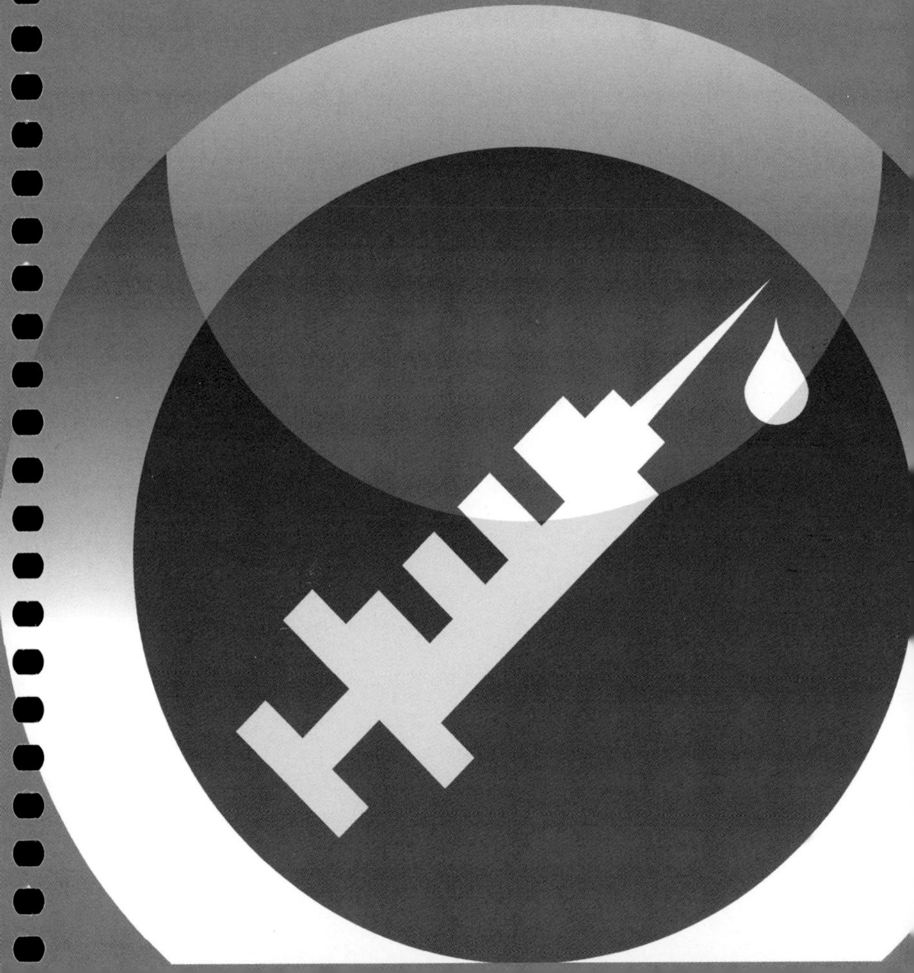

Chapter 1

Immunization Advocacy—Guidelines, Resources, and Tips

Recognizing the critical need for pharmacists to be involved in the practice and promotion of immunizations, in 1997 the American Pharmacists Association (APhA) Board of Trustees adopted a set of guidelines supporting immunization advocacy and delivery by pharmacists.[1] Regardless of geographic location and practice setting, pharmacists can be integrally involved in immunization advocacy by fulfilling at least one of three roles: educator, facilitator, and immunizer. In addition to supporting these roles, the guidelines provide a standard of practice for all pharmacists involved in immunizations. Table 1.1 summarizes the guidelines and provides tips for implementing them.

A 2002 position paper developed by the American College of Physicians–American Society of Internal Medicine Health and Public Policy Committee complements APhA's definitions of immunization advocacy roles for pharmacists.[2] It recognizes that pharmacists can help increase access to immunizations by providing immunization information, hosting immunization sites, and administering vaccines. In 2012, the U.S. Department of Health and Human Services (HHS) issued a letter addressed to pharmacists and community vaccinators, recognizing their efforts to increase immunization rates.[3] In this letter, HHS and CDC encourage continuation of these efforts. In summary, they request that pharmacists and other vaccinators increase public awareness of recommended vaccines, assess vaccine needs and offer the respective vaccines, recommend and offer vaccines intended for high-risk patients, document vaccine administration through immunization information systems and primary care providers, and collaborate with others such as state and local health departments, immunization coalitions, and medical providers to increase vaccine outreach efforts.

Vaccine advocacy by you and your pharmacy team can be a powerful means of increasing awareness of the importance of immunizations.

With the amount of attention that the media and the public have given to vaccine safety over the years, education as a component of advocacy is critical. A plethora of vaccine safety information, as well as misinformation, is available in print and on the Internet. Numerous false allegations misrepresenting vaccines have inundated the media in recent years. Most antivaccine websites reviewed in 2000 and 2003 claimed that vaccines were linked to conditions such as autism, asthma, diabetes, immune dysfunction, multiple sclerosis, neurologic disorders, and sudden infant death syndrome (SIDS).[4,5] An example of conflicting information regarding vaccine safety is the publication and subsequent retraction of Andrew Wakefield's controversial 1998 *Lancet* article linking the measles–mumps–rubella (MMR) vaccine to the development of autism.[6,7] A great deal of time and resources were devoted to disproving the false accusations and dispelling the myths spread by the media and the public as a result of this retracted publication.[7]

Recent studies have shown that parents continue to have concerns about the safety of vaccines and the risk for autism.[8,9] Nevertheless, most of the parents surveyed said they were following their health care providers' recommendations. Health care providers were deemed to be the most important source of vaccine information; media influence was ranked as the least important.[8] Unfortunately, the findings were different in a survey of parents who chose not to conform to routine vaccine recommendations.[10] These parents relied primarily on books or Internet sources when deciding to delay vaccination, to partially vaccinate, or to not vaccinate at all. A majority of these sources (59%) recommended nonconformity. In another survey in which 16% of parents intended to follow an alternative immunization schedule, parents who received information from friends, family, books, or their own professional background were more likely to report concerns such as overtaxing the immune system, aluminum or mercury exposure, and autism.[11] Given these findings, it is important to remember that personal advocacy by the pharmacist can have a profound impact on a patient's desire to be vaccinated.[12]

Your patients are likely to have questions about vaccines and vaccine safety. Approximately 60% of parents surveyed asked one to three questions pertaining to vaccines during routine appointments.[8] A review of 983 inquiries made to CDC's Immunization Safety Office (ISO) found that the most common topic was neurologic adverse events (17%). Other topics included autism and SIDS. The general public was the source of 19% of the inquiries to the ISO.[13] When patients or caregivers have safety concerns or questions about adverse events associated with vaccines, it is important to explain that the risk of serious adverse events is much lower than the risk associated with the vaccine-preventable disease. If a patient approaches you with safety concerns, you should check the source of that patient's information. Help your patients evaluate and understand the evidence on which the information is based, and guide them to credible scientific facts. The American Academy of Pediatrics has compiled a comprehensive list of studies that address the safety and efficacy of vaccines, accessible at www.aap.org/immunization/families/faq/vaccinestudies.pdf.

The following are additional examples of Web sources of reliable vaccine safety information:[14]

- Centers for Disease Control and Prevention, Vaccine Safety—www.cdc.gov/vaccinesafety
- Immunization Action Coalition, Vaccine Safety—www.immunize.org/safety/
- Institute of Medicine (IOM) Immunization Safety Review reports—www.iom.edu/Reports.aspx?Activity=%7B43C096A7-F094-43D0-985A-B6BF561A7C5D%7D&Date=more
- Institute for Vaccine Safety, Johns Hopkins Bloomberg School of Public Health—www.vaccinesafety.edu
- Minnesota Department of Health, Vaccine Safety—www.health.state.mn.us/divs/idepc/immunize/safety/index.html
- U.S. Department of Health and Human Services, vaccines.gov, Safety—vaccines.gov/basics/safety/index.html
- Children's Hospital of Philadelphia Vaccine Education Center, Vaccine Safety FAQs—www.chop.edu/service/vaccine-education-center/vaccine-safety/
- World Health Organization (WHO), Global Vaccine Safety—www.who.int/vaccine_safety/en/

In addition, the Immunization Action Coalition provides a list of websites and books that you can recommend to your patients and caregivers who are in search of reliable immunization information, at www.immunize.org/vaccine-safety-resources.pdf.

There are numerous opportunities to be involved in immunization advocacy at your practice site and in your community. The extent of your immunization activities is governed by your state's pharmacy laws and regulations. Regardless, you must ultimately decide how much time and energy you are willing and able to dedicate to the reduction and elimination of vaccine-preventable diseases. The suggestions provided in Table 1.1 and the activities described in the following chapters will help guide your immunization-related endeavors.

References

1. American Pharmacists Association. Guidelines for Pharmacy-Based Immunization Advocacy. Adopted August 1997. www.pharmacist.com/guidelines-pharmacy-based-immunization-advocacy. Accessed September 1, 2014.
2. American College of Physicians–American Society of Internal Medicine. Pharmacist scope of practice. *Ann Intern Med.* 2002;136:79–85.
3. U.S. Department of Health and Human Services. Letter to pharmacists and community vaccinators. June 26, 2012. www.nabp.net/news/assets/CDC_Letter_June_26_2012.pdf. Accessed September 1, 2014.
4. Zimmerman RK, Wolfe RM, Fox DE, et al. Vaccine criticism on the World Wide Web. *J Med Internet Res.* 2005;7(2):e17. www.jmir.org/2005/2/e17/. Accessed September 1, 2014.
5. Wolfe RM, Sharp LK, Lipsky MS. Content and design attributes of antivaccination web sites. *JAMA.* 2002;287:3245–8.
6. Editors of the Lancet. Retraction—ileal-lymphoid-nodular hyperplasia, non-specific colitis, and pervasive developmental disorder in children. *Lancet.* 2010;375:445.
7. Poland GA, Spier R. Fear, misinformation, and innumerates: how the Wakefield paper, the press, and advocacy groups damaged the public health [editorial]. *Vaccine.* 2010;28:2361–2.
8. Kennedy A, Basket M, Sheedy K. Vaccine attitudes, concerns, and information sources reported by parents of young children: results from the 2009 HealthStyles Survey. *Pediatrics.* 2011;127:S92–S99.
9. Freed GI, Clark SJ, Butchart AT, et al. Parental vaccine safety concerns in 2009. *Pediatrics.* 2010;125:654–9.
10. Brunson EK. The impact of social networks on parents' vaccination decisions. *Pediatrics.* 2013;131(5):e1397–e1404. http://pediatrics.aappublications.org/content/early/2013/04/10/peds.2012-2452.full.pdf. Accessed September 1, 2014.

11. Wheeler M, Buttenheim AM. Parental vaccine concerns, information source, and choice of alternative immunization schedules. *Hum Vaccin Immunother.* 2013;9(8):1782–1789. www.ncbi.nlm.nih.gov/pmc/articles/PMC3906282/. Accessed September 1, 2014.
12. Weitzel KW, Goode JR. Implementation of a pharmacy-based immunization program in a supermarket chain. *J Am Pharm Assoc.* 2000;40:252–6.
13. Miller E, Batten B, Hampton L, et al. Tracking vaccine-safety inquiries to detect signals and monitor public concerns. *Pediatrics.* 2011;127:S87–S91.
14. Pharmacy-Based Immunization Delivery: A National Certificate Program for Pharmacists. 11th ed. Washington, DC: American Pharmacists Association; 2009.

Table 1.1

Guidelines and Implementation Tips for Pharmacy-Based Immunization Advocacy and Delivery

1 Prevention

Protect your patient's health by being a vaccine advocate.

- Educate your patients and caregivers regarding the impact of disease and the importance of prevention.
- If you are not able to administer vaccines, facilitate the opportunity for others to do so by allowing them to vaccinate at your practice site.
- If you are able to administer vaccines, immunize as many patients as possible in accordance with your state practice act.

Focus your efforts on the most significant and detrimental vaccine-preventable diseases.

- Identify which vaccine-preventable diseases are most prominent in your community and which ones are known to cause the most morbidity and mortality (e.g., influenza, pneumococcal disease, hepatitis A and B, herpes zoster, meningococcal disease). Either immunize against these diseases or encourage your patients at risk for these diseases to be immunized.

continued on page 8

Table 1.1

continued from page 7

Routinely determine the immunization status of your patients, and refer as appropriate.

- Ask to see your patients' immunization records.
- When performing a medication therapy review, be sure to ask about previous vaccines received.
- When reconciling medications in the health-system environment, include vaccine history in this process.
- If you are not able to provide the vaccines they need, refer patients to a provider who can.

Identify your high-risk patients who are in need of specific vaccines.

- Recognize procedures, medications, and diagnoses most common in patients in need of vaccines. Examples include diabetes, human immunodeficiency virus (HIV) infection, and heart, lung, kidney, and liver disease.
- Check these high-risk patients against the immunization schedule for vaccines that might be indicated for adults on the basis of medical and other indications.
- Recognize the vaccines required in children and adolescents for school or college entry.
- Use the most up-to-date schedules to determine the vaccines your high-risk patients need.

Protect yourself from disease and infection.

- Be sure you are current on all the vaccines required for health care providers (see Chapter 17).
- Practice good hand washing and hygiene measures.

continued on page 9

2 Partnership

Partner with your community and other health care providers to promote and deliver vaccines.

- Support the goals and efforts of your local and state health departments.
- Collaborate with your health departments and prescribers within your community.
- Assist your patients in maintaining their medical homes and continuity of care, which should include routine vaccinations.
- Report vaccines administered to your patients' primary care providers and to immunization registries, as applicable.
- During medication reconciliation or the medication therapy review process, ensure that patients in hospital, institutional, and long-term care settings receive their needed vaccinations.

3 Quality

Before administering vaccines, receive proper education and training.

- Receive education that includes epidemiology, vaccine characteristics and contraindications, injection technique, emergency response, and patient consultation.
- Be evaluated to ensure that you are able to address or perform these immunization-related skills.

Keep your vaccine knowledge up-to-date.

- Join immunization-related electronic mailing lists.
- Receive continuing pharmacy education on vaccine topics.
- Refer to current immunization schedules and reference materials.

4 Documentation

Maintain accurate and complete immunization records for your patients.

- Whether you are using an electronic or a paper-based system, be sure to record all immunizations provided to your patients.

continued on page 10

Table 1.1

continued from page 9

- Provide your patients with their own immunization records, or offer to complete their records if they have them available.

Report vaccine adverse events.

- Inform your patient's primary care provider if the patient experiences an adverse event as a result of a vaccine you administered.
- Complete the appropriate documentation in accordance with the Vaccine Adverse Event Reporting System (VAERS), which can be found at http://vaers.hhs.gov.

5 Empowerment

Educate your patients about immunizations while respecting their rights as patients.

- Provide information to health care providers, employers, and your community to encourage the appropriate use of vaccines.
- Educate your patients and caregivers about the importance of vaccines in terms they can understand.
- Provide patient education materials, such as vaccine information statements, and document the provision of such materials.

Source: Reference 1.

Chapter 2

Active Involvement as an Immunization and Public Health Provider

Being recognized as an immunization provider is an opportunity that should not be overlooked. Through involvement in immunization activities, pharmacists can contribute to population-based care and public health initiatives.[1] The National Vaccine Advisory Committee's 2013 Standards for Adult Immunization Practice note that pharmacists are integral to increasing vaccination rates for adults.[2] Collaboration and partnership among immunization stakeholders are encouraged in these standards. Collaboration is a key component of the "immunization neighborhood"—a term coined by APhA to describe a concept involving "collaboration, coordination, and communication among immunization stakeholders, with the goal of meeting the immunization needs of patients and protecting the community from vaccine-preventable diseases."[3] Awards recognizing activities essential to immunization neighborhoods have been presented by the National Adult and Influenza Immunization Summit.[4] Joining an association, coalition, or advocacy group is the first step toward achieving nationally recognized immunization goals. The next step is active participation.

State Pharmacy Associations

Active involvement as an immunization provider begins with your state pharmacy association. The degree to which you can engage in the provision of immunizations is determined by your state practice act and legislation. Through involvement in your state pharmacy association, you can have an impact on professional practice and immunization activities in your state. If you want to secure your ability to provide the immunizations that your community needs, become an active member of your state association. Contact information for your state can be found on the National Alliance of State Pharmacy Associations website (www.naspa.us).

Immunization Coalitions

Immunization coalitions exist on both the national and state levels. These coalitions are made up of community activists and health professionals in the public and private sectors. The goals of coalition members are to improve immunization rates, advocate change, raise awareness about the importance of immunizations, and educate providers and the public regarding immunizations and preventive health measures. Often, coalitions partner with non-immunization groups to better reach members of the community and provide outreach. As a pharmacist involved in a coalition, you will serve as an expert on policy and practice issues that affect the pharmacy profession. Such interaction with other members of the coalition can help facilitate physician collaboration for your pharmacy-based service.[5] You may also be involved in planning and implementing community events. Such an opportunity serves to promote both immunizations and the service you offer.[6]

Activities of immunization coalitions

- Offer public speaking events and educational lectures
- Create educational materials for providers and the public
- Provide support for immunization registries
- Develop marketing campaigns
- Support each other's efforts and share a vision
- Advance the research efforts of individuals and groups
- Share information and keep each other informed

Roles for pharmacists in immunization coalitions[5]

- Chairing a committee
- Working with others to develop standing order templates
- Encouraging student pharmacists to participate in coalition activities
- Promoting vaccinations for health care personnel
- Providing pharmacy-specific messaging and marketing materials
- Updating members on pharmacy-specific issues
- Relaying specific examples of pharmacist–patient encounters

Numerous states encourage pharmacist involvement in their coalitions and offer a wide array of activities for pharmacists.[5] To find a coalition near you, go to the directory of immunization coalitions, searchable by state, at www.izcoalitions.org.

The Medical Reserve Corps

The Medical Reserve Corps (MRC) is a volunteer organization for medical and public health professionals. The MRC offers unique opportunities for pharmacists. As an MRC volunteer, you would primarily be involved in emergency preparedness in your community. Mass vaccine administration and medication dispensing are often emphasized in emergency planning activities. To meet federal compliance requirements for incident preparedness funding, the MRC offers National Incident Management System training so that volunteers are prepared to respond to and recover from emergency incidents.[7]

In emergency situations, MRC volunteers may be deployed locally or federally.[8] During non-emergencies, pharmacists may have the opportunity through their MRC unit to participate in public health initiatives such as mass immunization clinics and health fairs. During pandemics, pharmacist volunteers with expertise in immunizations can be an invaluable resource, providing educational outreach and assisting with mass immunization initiatives.[9] During the 2009 outbreak of the H1N1 virus, the MRC developed many educational initiatives for both providers and the public.[10] Public service announcements were created to guide communities' planning and preparedness efforts. Working in conjunction with their health departments, local MRC units organized immunization clinics to meet the vaccination needs of their communities.[9] A pandemic influenza planning guide is available for MRC units.[11] To find an MRC unit in your area, go to www.medicalreservecorps.gov/FindMRC.

Health Departments

State and county health departments also offer collaborative opportunities to promote immunization activities. Some offer immunization training programs for medical professionals. As a pharmacist, you would be useful as a faculty member for such programs. Both state and local health departments typically have a variety of resources specific to immunization administration in their areas. Health departments play a vital role during public health emergencies and pandemics. Responsible for vaccine distribution, health departments served as the primary resource to meet the mass vaccination needs during the 2009 H1N1 outbreak.[9,12] Pharmacies were included in the distribution process.[12,13] The health department in Palm Beach County, Florida, collaborated with a pharmacy–supermarket chain to develop a Flu Readiness Initiative.[14] This initiative, launched just before the 2009 H1N1 outbreak, included the timely distribution of more than 200,000 educational cards about the flu in 250 pharmacies and pharmacy-based health clinics throughout the county. In addition, the health department released approximately 12% of its 2009 H1N1 vaccine allocation to community pharmacies to increase vaccine access. Such collaboration can extend the reach of pharmacists' immunization efforts.

The following sites list contact information for state health departments and programs:

- www.immunize.org/states/
- www.cdc.gov/mmwr/international/relres.html

Immunizations for Those in Need

Pharmacists may also be relied upon to advocate and provide immunizations to those most in need, in settings such as the following:[9]

- Homeless shelters
- Community health centers
- Free or reduced-cost community clinics
- Recuperative care facilities
- Medical service trips (within the United States and abroad)
- Disaster relief efforts

For nearly two decades, pharmacists have been engaged in the delivery of immunizations to medically underserved populations. The Pharmacy Immunization Project (PIP), which began in 1995 in West Virginia, was based on a collaborative model between county health department nurses and independent pharmacies to improve immunization rates among underserved children.[15] Seven pharmacists were integrally involved in facilitating the provision of immunizations to children and adults. In the state of New York, the influenza vaccination educational efforts of pharmacists in a rural health clinic in 1999 led to a 26% increase in vaccination rates.[16] Direct mailings and clinic posters were used by the pharmacists to encourage vaccination. After Hurricane Katrina's 2005 devastation of New Orleans, pharmacists were actively involved in managing the vaccine supply during evacuee operations.[17] In 2009, a study involving the use of an immunization needs questionnaire found the role of a pharmacist immunizer to be key to increasing vaccination rates in underserved patients at a primary health care center in Pittsburgh.[18] Recently, immunization training has been recommended as one of several emergency preparedness measures for pharmacists.[19]

Liability Protections during Volunteer Activities

There are abundant opportunities for pharmacists to participate in immunization activities beyond their daily practice routines. Often, these involve serving in a volunteer capacity to meet a public health need. If you wish to engage in such activities, certain legal protections and scope of practice parameters need to be taken into consideration. For instance, if you are planning to provide immunizations during mass immunization clinics under the auspices of another organization, you will want to ensure that the standing orders and protocols include pharmacists. If you are traveling to a state to assist with disaster relief or a medical mission and you are not licensed in that state, you should contact that state's board of pharmacy to inquire about a temporary license transfer.[20] If you are going abroad, you should determine the regulations and scope of pharmacy practice in the specific location.[9] Often, the scope of practice for pharmacists in the United States applies in international locations.

During emergencies, immunity from civil liability may be granted by the state or covered under the U.S. Public Readiness and Emergency Preparedness (PREP) Act.[9] The PREP Act was amended in 2009 to cover pandemic countermeasures.[21] As a volunteer, especially in nonemergency situations, you will want to have your own professional liability insurance. This is also the case if you are affiliated with a for-profit entity or receive compensation for the services you provide.[22] Regardless of the circumstance, you should always operate strictly within your scope of practice and the standard of care expected of you as a pharmacist.

References

1. Stergachis A. APhA-APRS Association Report: promoting the pharmacist's role in public health. *J Am Pharm Assoc.* 2006;46:311–3.

2. National Vaccine Advisory Committee. Update on the National Vaccine Advisory Committee Standards for Adult Immunization Practice. September 10, 2013. www.hhs.gov/nvpo/nvac/reports/nvacstandards.pdf. Accessed September 1, 2014.

3. Tanzi MG. It takes a village: NVAC standards emphasize importance of immunization neighborhood. American Pharmacists Association Special Immunization Section. March 1, 2014. www.pharmacist.com/it-takes-village-nvac-standards-emphasize-importance-immunization-neighborhood. Accessed September 1, 2014.

4. National Adult and Influenza Immunization Summit. Immunization Excellence Awards. www.izsummitpartners.org/immunization-excellence-awards/. Accessed September 1, 2014.

5. Goad JA. Collaborative practice for pharmacy-based immunization. *Pharmacy Today.* October 2007:77–91.

6. Ernst ME, Charlstrom CV, Currie JD, et al. Implementation of a community pharmacy-based influenza vaccination program. *J Am Pharm Assoc.* 1997;NS37:570–80.

7. Office of the Civilian Volunteer Medical Reserve Corps. NIMS Guidance. www.medicalreservecorps.gov/SearchFldr/NIMSGuidance. Accessed September 1, 2014.

8. Frasca DR. The Medical Reserve Corps as part of the federal medical and public health response in disaster settings. *Biosecur Bioterror.* 2010;8:265–71.

9. Angelo LB, Maffeo CM. Local and global volunteer opportunities for pharmacists to contribute to public health. *Int J Pharm Pract.* 2011;19:206–13.

10. Office of the Civilian Volunteer Medical Reserve Corps. Medical Reserve Corps units and H1N1 influenza-related activities—September 2009. www.medicalreservecorps.gov/file/SwineFlu/MRC_Units_H1N1_Flu_Activities.pdf. Accessed September 1, 2014.

11. Office of the Civilian Volunteer Medical Reserve Corps. Guide to pandemic influenza planning for MRC units. www.medicalreservecorps.gov/file/MRC-PandemicFluPlanning-Final.pdf. Accessed September 1, 2014.

12. Centers for Disease Control and Prevention. H1N1 flu allocation and distribution Q&A. www.cdc.gov/H1N1flu/vaccination/statelocal/centralized_distribution_qa.htm. Accessed September 1, 2014.

13. The Association of State and Territorial Health Officials. Operational framework for partnering with pharmacies for administration of 2009 H1N1 vaccine.

September 28, 2009. www.astho.org/Programs/Infectious-Disease/H1N1/OpFramework_Pharmacies_STHOs_FINAL/. Accessed September 1, 2104.

14. Rosenfeld LA, Etkind P, Grasso A, et al. Extending the reach: local health department collaboration with community pharmacies in Palm Beach County, Florida for H1N1 influenza pandemic response. *J Public Health Manag Pract* 2011;17(5):439–48.

15. Rosenbluth SA, Madhavan SS, Borker RD, et al. Pharmacy immunization partnerships: a rural model. *J Am Pharm Assoc.* 2001;41:100–7.

16. Van Amburgh JA, Waite NM, Hobson EH, et al. Improved influenza vaccination rates in a rural population as a result of a pharmacist-managed immunization campaign. *Pharmacotherapy.* 2001;21:1115–22.

17. Young D. Medical Reserve Corps pharmacists assist evacuees. *Am J Health Syst Pharm.* 2006;63:296,299–300,302.

18. Higginbotham S, Stewart A, Pfalzgraf A. Impact of pharmacist immunizer on adult immunization rates. *J Am Pharm Assoc.* 2012;52:367–71.

19. Woodard LJ, Bray BS, Williams D, et al. Call to action: integrating student pharmacists, faculty, and pharmacy practitioners into emergency preparedness and response. *J Am Pharm Assoc.* 2010;50:158–64.

20. National Association of Boards of Pharmacy. NABP facilitates emergency pharmacist license transfer medication distribution efforts to aid Hurricane Katrina victims. www.nabp.net/news/nabp-facilitates-emergency-pharmacist-license-transfer-medication-distribution-efforts-to-aid-hurricane-katrina-victims. Accessed September 1, 2014.

21. Pandemic influenza vaccines. Amendment to 42 USC § 247d-6d. http://edocket.access.gpo.gov/2009/E9-14948.htm. Accessed September 1, 2014.

22. Hodge JG, Gable LA, Cálves SH. Volunteer health professionals and emergencies: assessing and transforming the legal environment. *Biosecur Bioterror.* 2005;3:216–23.

Chapter 3

Staying Informed

The immunization field is constantly changing. New vaccines, formulations, and administration methods are continually under development. Guidelines and practice recommendations are routinely updated. Outbreaks and pandemics can occur without warning. As a health care provider involved in immunization delivery, it is your responsibility to keep up-to-date. The National Vaccine Advisory Committee's 2013 Standards for Adult Immunization Practice recommend that all immunization providers stay up-to-date and maintain their professional competencies regarding immunizations.[1]

Resources to Ensure Professional Competencies

You are busy and your time is valuable. You may not be able to routinely search for updated information on immunizations, so let the information come to you. A good place to start is to bookmark the following two websites on your computer:

- www.cdc.gov/vaccines
- www.immunize.org

Another easy way to keep up is to subscribe to electronic mailing lists from reputable sources (Table 3.1).[2] You can also subscribe to Really Simple Syndication (RSS) feeds, such as those offered by CDC at www2c.cdc.gov/podcasts/rss.asp, which will automatically download information to your computer or mobile device.

In addition to receiving routine updates electronically, there are other ways to learn about the latest developments in immunization practice. The following are some examples.

- The Advisory Committee on Immunization Practices (ACIP) meets at least three times a year to discuss changes in vaccine recommendations and develop new recommendations. The meeting agendas, minutes, and presentation slides can be found at www.cdc.gov/vaccines/acip/meetings/meetings-info.html.

- Before each seasonal influenza season, the ACIP provides updated recommendations for the prevention and control of influenza ("Prevention and Control of Seasonal Influenza with Vaccines: Recommendations of the ACIP—U.S."). These can be found in the *Morbidity and Mortality Weekly Report (MMWR)* or on the CDC website at www.cdc.gov/vaccines/hcp/acip-recs/vacc-specific/flu.html.
- At the beginning of each year, updated immunization schedules are approved by the ACIP. To view and download these, go to www.cdc.gov/vaccines/schedules/index.html.
- CDC keeps track of vaccine shortages and delays and provides information on how to handle each situation. This information can be found at www.cdc.gov/vaccines/vac-gen/shortages/default.htm.
- CDC routinely creates podcasts and webcasts to relay important vaccine information. These can be viewed at www.cdc.gov/vaccines/ed/podcasts.htm and www.cdc.gov/vaccines/ed/courses.htm, respectively.
- CDC routinely updates its textbook *Epidemiology and Prevention of Vaccine-Preventable Diseases* (The Pink Book). It can be accessed free of charge at www.cdc.gov/vaccines/pubs/pinkbook/index.html.
- CDC posts a list of its partner websites, which contain a variety of resources for immunization providers. This is available at www.cdc.gov/vaccines/imz-managers/partners.html.
- CDC provides a variety of social media tools, available at www.cdc.gov/SocialMedia/index.html.
- CDC provides a free vaccine schedule app for iOS and Android devices, available at www.cdc.gov/vaccines/schedules/hcp/schedule-app.html.
- The APhA Immunization Center is located at www.pharmacist.com/immunization-center.
- APhA provides immunization updates as continuing pharmacy education (CPE) programs each year at the APhA Annual Meeting and Exposition and via online webinars. Webinar registration information can be found in the Immunization Center.
- CPE activities on immunization are routinely made available by APhA and other national and state pharmacy associations.

- Information on APhA's Pharmacy-Based Immunization Delivery: A National Certificate Program for Pharmacists can be found at www.pharmacist.com/apha-training-programs.

Keeping Up with Pandemics and Outbreaks

When an outbreak or pandemic occurs, patients, the community, and other health care providers will look to you for information. Fortunately, CDC and the World Health Organization (WHO) will take measures to track cases, deaths, and the overall situation. WHO has a website dedicated to tracking outbreaks on a global level (www.who.int/csr/outbreak network/en/). The disease tracking and outreach efforts of CDC and WHO were invaluable as reports of human cases of swine influenza A (H1N1) began to make headlines in the spring of 2009. Health care providers across the world were called upon to assist in infection control. Guidelines for managing the sick were developed and widely disseminated. Seasonal influenza and pneumococcal vaccine recommendations were revisited. New websites and numerous educational pieces and guidance documents for patients and providers were created. A variety of social media tools were developed by CDC, including social networking sites, online image sharing, and Twitter feeds.[3] Vaccine manufacturers and researchers increased their efforts to develop a vaccine against H1N1. Both nationally and internationally, communities were put on high alert. Although this situation came about unexpectedly, the leading immunization experts and organizations handled it in an outstanding and efficient manner.

In response to measles and mumps outbreaks in Ohio, on June 9, 2014, pharmacists were permitted to administer the MMR vaccine to patients 18 years of age and older pursuant to an emergency order signed by the governor.[4,5] To embrace this additional responsibility, not only would Ohio pharmacists need to institute a new protocol that includes MMR, established by a physician and approved by the board of pharmacy, they would also need to be prepared to educate about and administer the MMR vaccine.

Your regular efforts to keep up-to-date regarding immunization events and practices will provide you with ample opportunity to participate in managing emergency situations such as these.

References

1. National Vaccine Advisory Committee. Update on the National Vaccine Advisory Committee Standards for Adult Immunization Practice. September 10, 2013. www.hhs.gov/nvpo/nvac/reports/nvacstandards.pdf. Accessed September 6, 2014.
2. Gatewood S, Goode JR, Stanley D. Keeping up-to-date on immunizations: a framework and review for pharmacists. *J Am Pharm Assoc.* 2006;46:183–92.
3. Centers for Disease Control and Prevention. Social media at CDC. Novel H1N1 flu (swine flu). www.cdc.gov/socialmedia/campaigns/h1n1. Accessed October 11, 2009.
4. National Association of Boards of Pharmacy. Ohio pharmacists may now administer MMR vaccines. June 28, 2014. www.nabp.net/news/ohio-pharmacists-may-now-administer-mmr-vaccines. Accessed September 6, 2014.
5. Ohio State Board of Pharmacy. Pharmacists Can Now Administer the Measles, Mumps, and Rubella (MMR) Vaccine. June 9, 2014. www.pharmacy.ohio.gov/Pubs/NewsReleases.aspx. Accessed September 6, 2014.

Table 3.1

Electronic Mailing Lists for Immunization Providers

Immunization Action Coalition Express and other periodicals	Go to www.immunize.org/subscribe/ Select the items you would like to receive
APhA Immunizing Pharmacists News Mailing List	Go to www.pharmacist.com/node/26020?is_sso_called=1
CDC Email Updates	Go to https://service.govdelivery.com/accounts/USCDC/subscriber/new Select the items you would like to receive
CDC *Morbidity and Mortality Weekly Report*	Go to www.cdc.gov/mmwr/mmwrsubscribe.html Enter your email in the space provided and click "Submit"

Adapted from: Reference 2.

Chapter 4

Vaccine Supplies, Preparation, and Administration

Vaccine Supplies

Before you begin to administer vaccines, you will need to have a sufficient stock of supplies (Table 4.1). The supplies you will need to administer vaccines are the same regardless of whether your pharmacy has a separate area reserved for vaccine administration, with storage space for supplies, or an area with limited space in which a supply cart is used. Your supplies should include an emergency kit and an exposure control plan, which are further discussed in Chapters 15 and 17, respectively. The items listed in Table 4.1 are available from your wholesaler and medical supply companies. Please note the following when ordering supplies:

- Order a variety of needles and syringes to accommodate various patient sizes and different routes of administration.
- Have appropriate sizes of disposable gloves available for all those involved in immunizations.
- Preferably, use synthetic adhesive bandages and disposable gloves to avoid adverse reactions in patients allergic to latex.

The types of vaccines you will need to order and the quantity depend on your patient volume and demographics. Consider the ages of your patients, their chronic conditions, commonly used medications, and the routinely recommended immunizations that they will need. CDC recommends that providers order and stock enough vaccine to meet the needs of their patients—typically, enough to last 60 days, with a reorder threshold of 30 days.[1] An exception may be influenza vaccine, for which pre-orders are placed in the late spring or early summer in preparation for the upcoming influenza season. CDC advises providers not to order more vaccine than what they realistically need, to avoid vaccine expiration or unnecessary financial loss should vaccine storage be compromised.[1]

Table 4.2 lists contact information for vaccine manufacturers and device suppliers.[2] This is not an all-inclusive list; you may wish to work with your wholesalers to identify additional suppliers and manufacturers.

Injectable Vaccine Preparation

Two crucial elements of vaccine delivery are the preparation and the administration of the vaccine. Errors introduced during either of these activities could result in direct harm to the patient. Sterility, correct dose, and proper drug selection must all be ensured. Individuals involved in preparing and administering vaccines should have proper training and adequate practice. The individual's ability to successfully prepare and administer vaccines should be evaluated by an experienced immunizer before the individual is allowed to immunize a patient.

Before preparing the dose and administering the vaccine to the patient, you should always do the following:

- Select the appropriate syringe size.
- Select the appropriate needle gauge.
- Select the appropriate needle length.
- Check the vaccine name and contents.
- Check the expiration date.
- Double check the vaccine ordered for the patient.

Table 4.3 details the appropriate needle gauge and length for the patient by sex and weight.[3] The syringe size will be determined by the volume of vaccine needed. Use syringes that are calibrated in milliliters (mL) or cubic centimeters (cc) and in increments that will allow you to measure the correct dose.

Product packaging and form vary depending on the type of vaccine and the manufacturer. Many vaccines come as suspensions and simply need to be agitated before use. Others, however, require reconstitution with the diluent provided. Many vaccine manufacturers offer various packaging and size options from which you can choose. Single-dose vials, multidose vials, and prefilled syringes may be available. Some prefilled syringes come with needles; others do not. Check with your wholesaler or the manufacturer, or refer to the package insert to determine how the vaccine products you need are supplied. (See Chapter 19 for product information on commonly used products.)

The preparation process differs according to vaccine type, manufacturer, and product type (i.e., single-dose vials, multidose vials, prefilled syringes, lyophilized powder requiring reconstitution). Always refer to the vaccine's package insert for specific information on preparation of the vaccine. Tables 4.4 and 4.5 give step-by-step procedures for preparing vaccines that require reconstitution and those that exist as suspensions, respectively. The storage requirements for vaccines after they have been reconstituted can be found in Chapter 19.

Vaccine Administration

Intramuscular (IM) injection is the most common administration method for the vaccines that are available in the United States. As a general rule, inactivated vaccines are given via the IM route; meningococcal polysaccharide vaccine, which is administered subcutaneously, is the exception to this rule. Live attenuated vaccines, however, are injected subcutaneously or administered orally or intranasally. Chapter 19 provides the administration routes for commonly encountered vaccines. The techniques used to administer IM and subcutaneous injections differ slightly. As noted in Table 4.3, the needle lengths and gauges are different.[3] As depicted in Figure 4.1, IM injections should be administered at a 90° angle into the deltoid muscle, and subcutaneous injections should be administered at a 45° angle into the posterolateral aspect of the upper arm for adults and most children over the age of 36 months. When giving IM injections into the deltoid muscle, be sure to inject into the central and thickest portion of the muscle. Injecting too high has been associated with severe shoulder injuries (e.g., bursitis, tendonitis).[4] Subcutaneous injections given to infants less than 12 months of age should be administered into the fatty tissue over the anterolateral thigh muscle. IM injections given to children younger than 3 years of age should be administered into the anterolateral thigh muscle.[3,5] Pharmacists administering vaccines to young children should receive training and education beyond the information provided in this book.

Table 4.6 outlines the steps that should be followed during the administration process. It is important to practice both types of injections until you are comfortable with the process, ensuring that the vaccine is administered in the appropriate site and injury to the patient does not result.

There are three additional delivery methods for the influenza virus vaccine: intranasal, intradermal, and needle-free injection. The live attenuated influenza virus (LAIV) vaccine was approved for intranasal use in 2003, an intradermal formulation of the inactivated influenza vaccine was approved in May 2011, and a needle-free injection device for administration of the Afluria influenza vaccine was approved in August 2014.[6–8] Each of these has specific age limitations. Refer to Chapter 19 and the most current package insert for indications for use. The intradermal and needle-free injections can result in higher rates of local reactions (e.g., erythema, induration, pruritus) than IM injections, but these reactions tend to be transient and well tolerated.[9–14] Figures 4.2 and 4.3 depict the administration steps for the intranasal and intradermal influenza vaccines, respectively. Because the use of needle-free injection technology is more complex, with several different components to preparation and administration of the vaccine, pharmacists who choose to use this technology are encouraged to contact the device manufacturer for guidance and training (http://pharmajet.com).

Injectable vaccine preparation and administration pearls

- Maintain aseptic technique throughout.
- Aspiration, which is the act of pulling back on the plunger to check for blood before the injection is given, is no longer recommended.
- If the needle contacts bone during an intramuscular injection, the patient will not feel it. Simply pull back on the syringe until the needle resides in the deltoid muscle and proceed with the injection.
- When giving a subcutaneous injection, avoid excessive squeezing of the skin around the injection site while injecting the vaccine and withdrawing the needle. This could result in loss of vaccine through the hole created upon needle insertion. Waiting a couple seconds after injecting the vaccine before withdrawing the needle may also minimize loss of vaccine.

continued on page 27

Injectable vaccine preparation and administration pearls,
continued from page 26

- Never recap a needle once it has come into contact with a patient.
- Clean and sterilize the work space after an immunization is given.
- Wash your hands between patients.
- Although it is not required, wearing disposable gloves is recommended for both your safety and the patient's comfort. Gloves must be changed between patients.
- Document all immunizations given.

References

1. Centers for Disease Control and Prevention. Vaccine Storage and Handling Toolkit. May 2014. www.cdc.gov/vaccines/recs/storage/toolkit/. Accessed September 6, 2014.
2. American Pharmacists Association. Pharmacy-Based Immunization Delivery: A National Certificate Program for Pharmacists. 11th ed. Washington, DC: American Pharmacists Association; 2009.
3. Immunization Action Coalition. Administering vaccines: dose, route, site, and needle size. www.immunize.org/catg.d/p3085.pdf. Accessed September 6, 2014.
4. Foster SL, Davis MV. Vaccine administration: preventing serious shoulder injuries. *J Am Pharm Assoc.* 2013;53:102–3.
5. Minnesota Department of Health. Vaccine Administration: Guidelines for administering vaccines and handling vaccine reactions. July 2011. www.health.state.mn.us/divs/idepc/immunize/hcp/provguide/vaxadmin.pdf. Accessed September 14, 2014.
6. U.S. Food and Drug Administration. June 17, 2003 Approval Letter—Influenza Virus Vaccine Live, Intranasal. www.fda.gov/BiologicsBloodVaccines/Vaccines/ApprovedProducts/ucm123753.htm. Accessed September 14, 2014.
7. U.S. Food and Drug Administration. May 19, 2011 Approval Letter—Fluzone Intradermal. www.fda.gov/BiologicsBloodVaccines/Vaccines/ApprovedProducts/ucm255160.htm. Accessed September 14, 2014.
8. U.S. Food and Drug Administration. August 15, 2014 Approval Letter—Afluria. www.fda.gov/BiologicsBloodVaccines/Vaccines/ApprovedProducts/ucm410327.htm. Accessed September 14, 2014.
9. Frenck RW Jr, Belshe R, Brady RC, et al. Comparison of the immunogenicity and safety of a split-virion, inactivated, trivalent influenza vaccine (Fluzone®) administered by intradermal and intramuscular route in healthy adults. *Vaccine.* 2011;29(34):5666–74.

10. Gorse GJ, Falsey AR, Fling JA, et al. Intradermally-administered influenza virus vaccine is safe and immunogenic in healthy adults 18–64 years of age. *Vaccine.* 2013;31(19):2358–65.
11. Moro PL, Harrington T, Shimabukuro T, et al. Adverse events after Fluzone® Intradermal vaccine reported to the Vaccine Adverse Event Reporting System (VAERS), 2011–2013. *Vaccine.* 2013;31(43):4984–7.
12. Chi RC, Rock MT, Neuzil KM. Immunogenicity and safety of intradermal influenza vaccination in healthy older adults. *Clin Infect Dis.* 2010;50(10)1331–8.
13. Simon JK, Carter M, Pasetti MF, et al. Safety, tolerability, and immunogenicity of inactivated trivalent seasonal influenza vaccine administered with a needle-free disposable-syringe jet injector. *Vaccine.* 2011;29(51):9544–50.
14. McAllister L, Anderson J, Werth K, et al. Needle-free jet injection for administration of influenza vaccine: a randomised non-inferiority trial. *Lancet.* 2014;384(9944):674–81.
15. Centers for Disease Control and Prevention. *Epidemiology and Prevention of Vaccine-Preventable Diseases.* Atkinson W, Wolfe S, Hamborsky J, eds. 12th ed., 2nd printing. Washington, DC: Public Health Foundation; 2012.

Table 4.1

Vaccine Administration Supply List

- Vaccine for administration
- Vaccine diluent, as needed to reconstitute lyophilized powders
- Needles and syringes of appropriate sizes
- Absorbent pad to cover your workspace
- Adhesive bandages
- Cotton balls or gauze pads
- Alcohol swabs
- Disposable synthetic gloves
- Hand sanitizer, if applicable
- Sharps disposal container
- Biohazard disposal bag
- Exposure control plan
- Emergency kit (e.g., epinephrine, epinephrine dosing chart, diphenhydramine, blood pressure cuffs, stethoscope, CPR barriers or face shields)

Table 4.2

Vaccine Manufacturers and Immunization Device Suppliers

Company	Website	Telephone Number
Becton, Dickinson and Company	http://catalog.bd.com/nexus-ecat/categories	201-847-6800
Berna Products (Crucell Vaccines, Inc.)	www.bernaproducts.com	800-533-5899
CSL	www.cslbiotherapies.com	888-435-8633
Emergent BioSolutions	www.emergentbiosolutions.com	800-441-4225
GlaxoSmithKline	www.gsk.com	888-825-5249
GRP & Associates, Inc.	www.sharpsdisposal.com/	800-207-0976
MedImmune	www.medimmune.com	301-398-0000
Merck Vaccine Division	www.merckvaccines.com	877-829-6372
Novartis Vaccines	www.novartisvaccines.com	877-683-473
Pfizer	www.pfizerpro.com/vaccinesordering	800-505-4426
Pharmajet	http://pharmajet.com/	888-900-4321
Protein Sciences Corporation	www.proteinsciences.com/	800-488-7099
Retractable Technologies, Inc.	www.vanishpoint.com	888-703-1010
Sanofi Pasteur	www.sanofipasteur.us	800-822-2463
Sharps Compliance, Inc.	www.sharpsinc.com	800-772-5657
Stericycle	www.stericycle.com/sharps-disposal	866-783-9816

Adapted from: Reference 2.

Table 4.3

Appropriate Needle Gauge and Length by Injection Type

Injection Type	Needle Gauge	Needle Length
Subcutaneous	23–25	⅝ inch
Intramuscular	22–25	
Men and women <60 kg (<130 lb)		⅝–1 inch[a]
Women 60–90 kg (130–200 lb)		1–1½ inches
Women >90 kg (>200 lb)		1½ inches
Men 60–118 kg (130–260 lb)		1–1½ inches
Men >118 kg (>260 lb)		1½ inches
Children		⅝–1¼ inches[b]

[a] *If a ⅝-inch needle is used, it must be inserted at a 90° angle, with the skin stretched tight so that it extends beyond the subcutaneous tissue.*

[b] *Varies according to age and anatomic site of administration.*

Adapted from: Reference 3.

Table 4.4

Dose Preparation Checklist for Vials Requiring Reconstitution

- ☐ Check expiration dates on vials of lyophilized powder and diluent.
- ☐ Remove plastic caps from both vials.
- ☐ Swab top of vials with alcohol swab in one smooth motion.
- ☐ Pull back on the syringe to draw up air equivalent to the amount of diluent needed.
- ☐ Insert the needle into the vial of diluent.
- ☐ Depress the plunger to inject air into the vial.
- ☐ Invert the vial and withdraw the diluent.
- ☐ Remove any large air bubbles.
- ☐ Remove the needle from the vial.
- ☐ Insert the needle into the vial containing the lyophilized powder.
- ☐ Depress the plunger to inject the diluent into the vial.
- ☐ Remove the needle from the vial.
- ☐ Mix the diluent and powder until it forms a cloudy mixture free of particles.
- ☐ Replace the needle used for reconstituting with an unused needle, if applicable.[a]
- ☐ Pull back on the syringe to draw up air equivalent to the amount of vaccine needed.
- ☐ Insert the needle into the vial.
- ☐ Depress the plunger to inject air into the vial.
- ☐ Invert the vial and withdraw the proper amount of vaccine.
- ☐ Remove any large air bubbles.
- ☐ Remove the needle from the vial.
- ☐ Administer the vaccine to the patient (see Table 4.6).

[a]*Although the CDC states that changing the needle after reconstituting and before administering the vaccine is not necessary unless the needle has been contaminated or damaged,[15] some practitioners and company policies prefer that the needle be changed. If this is the case, simply replace the needle used for reconstituting with an unused needle and proceed with vaccine administration. If the syringe is equipped with a safety device that does not allow for needle removal, a new syringe will need to be used. When this is the case, consider using a less expensive syringe and needle for reconstitution.*

Table 4.5

Dose Preparation Checklist for Single-Dose and Multidose Vials Containing a Suspension

- ☐ Check expiration date on the vial.
- ☐ Shake the vial.
- ☐ Check for a cloudy mixture without precipitants.
- ☐ Remove plastic cap from the vial.
- ☐ Swab top of the vial with alcohol swab in one smooth motion.
- ☐ Pull back on the syringe to draw up air equivalent to the amount of vaccine needed.
- ☐ Insert the needle into the vial.
- ☐ Depress the plunger to inject air into the vial.
- ☐ Invert the vial and withdraw the proper amount of vaccine.
- ☐ Remove any large air bubbles.
- ☐ Remove the needle from the vial.
- ☐ Administer the vaccine to the patient (see Table 4.6).

Table 4.6

Vaccine Administration Checklist

- ☐ Select the proper injection site.
- ☐ Prepare the injection site by wiping with alcohol in a circular motion.
- ☐ Allow the alcohol to dry.
- ☐ Stabilize the patient during injection.
- ☐ Hold the syringe near the hub.
- ☐ Insert the needle to the hub in a smooth, coordinated motion at the appropriate angle.
- ☐ Inject the vaccine by applying steady pressure on the plunger.
- ☐ Withdraw the needle in the same smooth motion and angle in which it was inserted.
- ☐ Activate the safety device on the syringe.[a]
- ☐ Dispose of the syringe and needle in the sharps container immediately.
- ☐ Provide injection site care.

[a]Some syringes have safety devices that can be activated while the needle is still in the patient. Check with the syringe manufacturer to confirm the appropriate activation technique.

Figure 4.1

Intramuscular and Subcutaneous Injection Sites for Adults and Children over the Age of 36 Months

Intramuscular (IM) injection angle and site

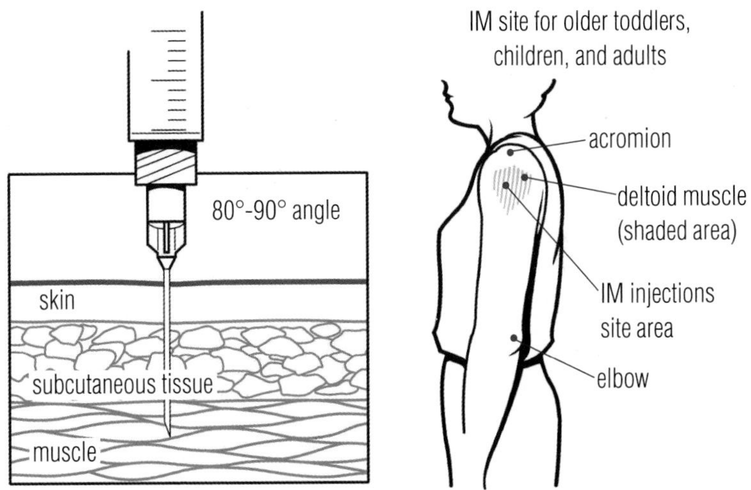

Subcutaneous (SQ) injection angle and site

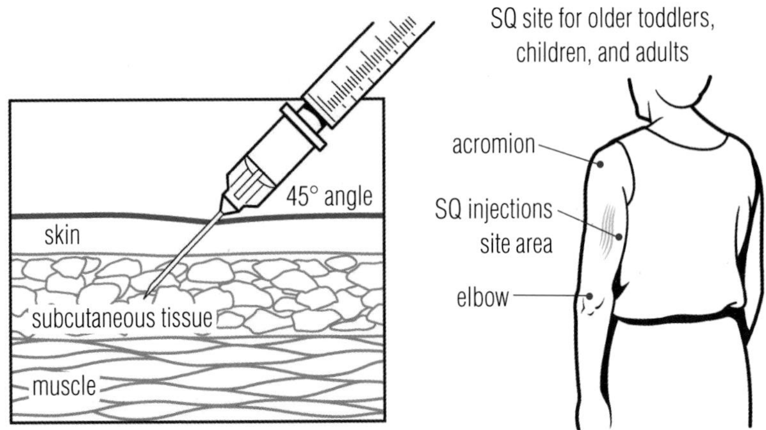

Used with permission of Minnesota Department of Health Immunization Program.

Figure 4.2

Intranasal Influenza Vaccine (FluMist) Administration

1

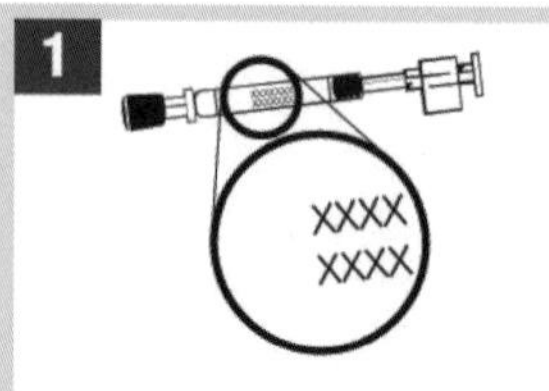

Check expiration date. Product must be used before the date on sprayer label.

2

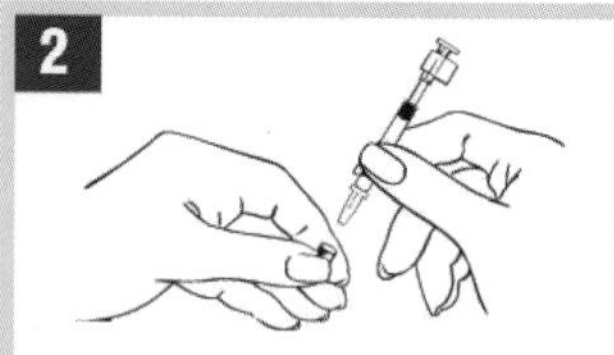

Remove rubber tip protector. Do not remove dose-divider clip at the other end of the sprayer.

3

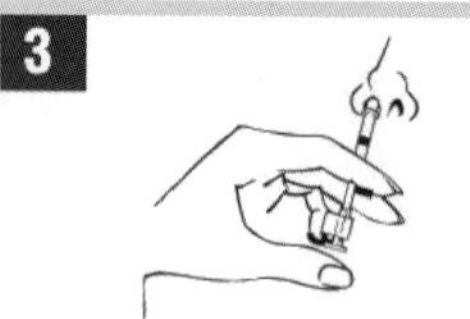

With the patient in an upright position, place the tip just inside the nostril to ensure FluMist® is delivered into the nose.

4

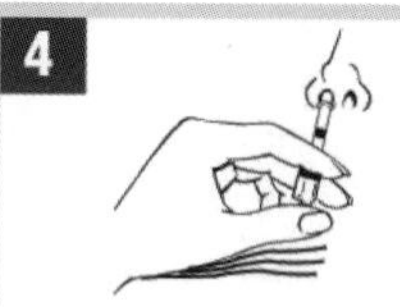

With a single motion, depress plunger **as rapidly as possible** until the dose-divider clip prevents you from going further.

5

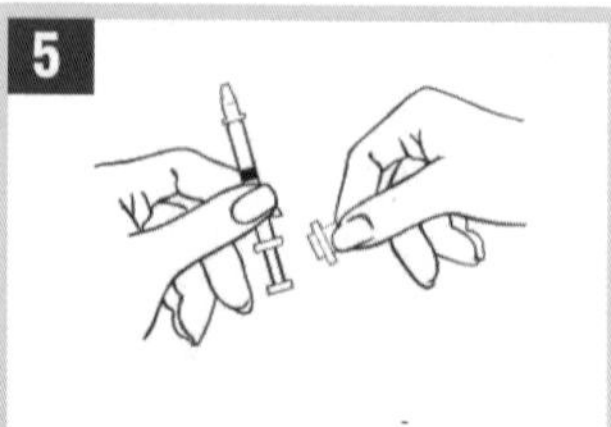

Pinch and remove the dose-divider clip from plunger.

6

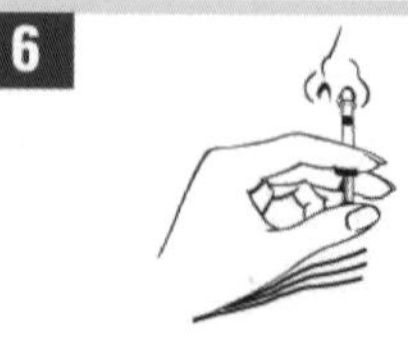

Place the tip just inside the other nostril and with a single motion, depress plunger **as rapidly as possible** to deliver remaining vaccine.

Used with permission of MedImmune.

Figure 4.3

Intradermal Influenza Vaccine (Fluzone) Administration

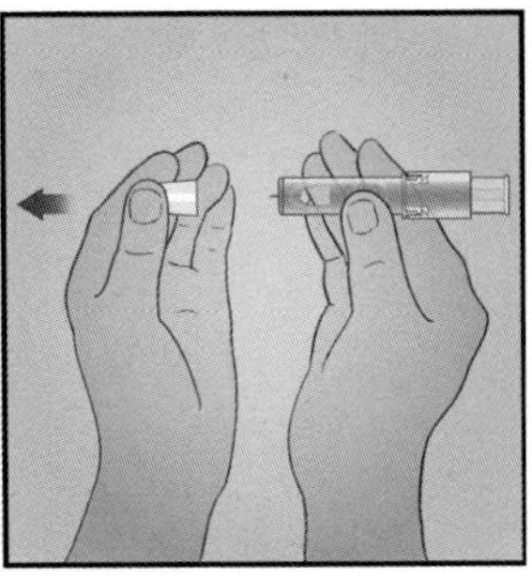

1. Remove needle cap.

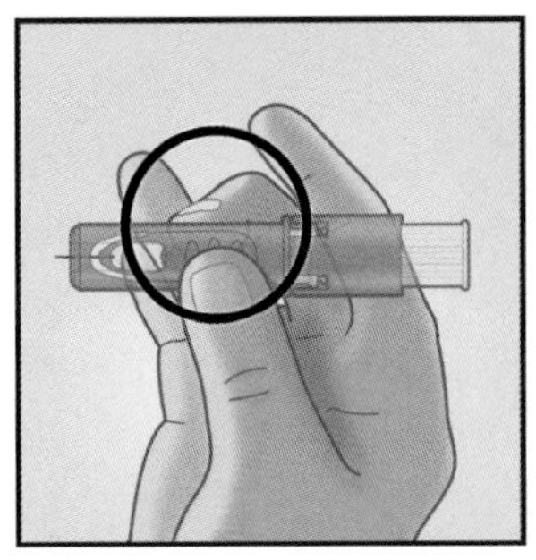

2. Hold microinjection system between thumb and middle finger.

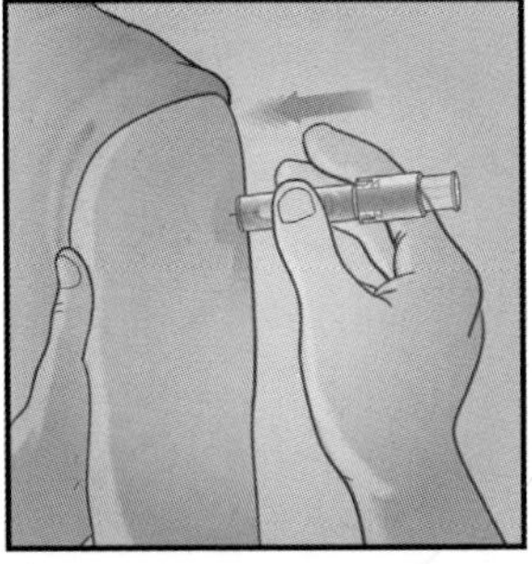

3. Insert needle rapidly in the area of the deltoid muscle, perpendicular to the skin.

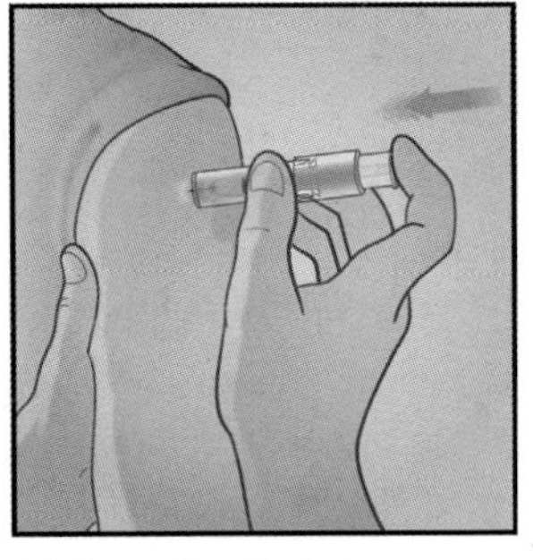

4. Inject using the index finger.

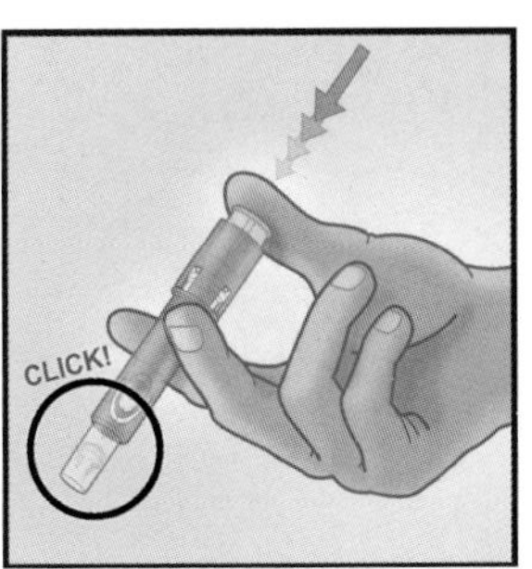

5. Remove needle from skin and activate needle shield by pushing firmly on plunger.

Used with permission of Sanofi Pasteur.

Chapter 5

Vaccine Storage and Handling

Each vaccine has specific storage and handling criteria. Procedures for complying with these criteria should be implemented before your first vaccine order is made. It is your responsibility and the responsibility of your staff to ensure that the integrity of your vaccine supply is maintained and patient safety is not compromised. The recommendations in this chapter provide detailed steps to follow to ensure safe vaccine storage and handling.

Vaccine storage conditions must be maintained from the moment vaccines are manufactured until they are administered to the patient. The "cold chain" is the term used to describe the process of maintaining proper storage conditions and temperatures.[1] Individuals and processes involved at each link in the chain are responsible for ensuring that storage temperatures are maintained (Figure 5.1).[1] Remember that vaccine stability is only as good as the weakest link in the chain. Exposure to extreme heat or cold may damage vaccines, rendering them ineffective. When vaccines are transported from one location to the next, an insulated container or refrigerated truck should be used. Delivery to the pharmacy should occur only when trained personnel can accept the shipment. Immediately upon arrival of vaccines, the temperature indicators and cold packs in the shipping case should be checked. Then, the vaccines should be unpacked and placed in the appropriate storage units in the pharmacy. Guidance for maintaining the cold chain while transporting vaccines to off-site clinics is addressed in Chapter 13.

Recommendations for Vaccine Storage Equipment[1,2]

- Use standalone refrigerator and freezer units. If a combination unit is used, then only refrigerated vaccines should be stored in the refrigerator compartment, away from the cold air outlet between the refrigerator and freezer;

continued on page 38

Recommendations for Vaccine Storage Equipment,
continued from page 37

frozen vaccines should be in a separate unit. Note that dormitory-style units are not recommended and are prohibited for Vaccines for Children (VFC) program providers.

- Allow for adequate space and ventilation around the units. Units should be at least 4 inches (10 cm) from the wall and 1 to 2 inches (2.5 to 5 cm) above the floor.
- Routinely check that the units seal properly when the doors are closed.
- When using a new unit, monitor temperatures twice daily for at least 1 week to establish a stable operating temperature before storing vaccines in the unit.
- Use water bottles in the refrigerator and frozen coolant packs in the freezer both to stabilize temperatures and to prevent placement of vaccine in the doors, along the walls, or on the bottom of the units.
- Do not store food or beverages for consumption in units containing vaccines.
- Remove the deli, fruit, and vegetable drawers. Do not store vaccines where these drawers were located; rather, use this space for water bottles.
- Maintain the refrigerator temperature at 2–8°C (35–46°F), with an average of 5°C (40°F).
- Maintain the freezer temperature at –15°C (5°F) or colder, but not below –50°C (–58°F).
- Keep the units clean, both inside and out, and perform routine maintenance on the units.
- Post a "Do Not Unplug" sign next to the electrical outlets.
- Identify and maintain a backup storage unit that can be used in the event of power or unit failure.
- Keep a logbook for equipment (e.g., serial numbers, dates of installation, maintenance, repair).
- In the event of refrigerator or freezer failure, follow these steps:
    - Place the vaccines in an alternative location that meets the temperature requirements.
    - Identify the exposed vaccines, mark them as "Exposed" or "Do Not Use," and separate them from the undamaged stock.
    - Note the refrigerator or freezer temperature at the time of failure, and contact the vaccine manufacturers or your state health department to determine your next course of action.

Recommendations for Thermometers and Temperature Monitoring[1,2]

- Use only calibrated thermometers with a Certificate of Traceability and Calibration Testing (also known as Report of Calibration); check with the thermometer manufacturer to determine when recalibration is necessary.
- Use thermometers with high accuracy readings: +/–1°F (+/–0.5°C).
- Use a digital thermometer with a detachable probe that is kept in a glycol-filled bottle.
- Keep a monitor with the temperature reading outside each storage unit. The device should provide continuous monitoring, with an alarm for temperatures out of range.
- Read and document the temperature for each unit at least twice each workday, and record the minimum and maximum temperatures once each day.
- Post temperature logs on the refrigerator and freezer for recording temperatures twice a day. Include contact information for notifying the appropriate individual if the temperature is out of range. Sample logs can be obtained from the Immunization Action Coalition (www.immunize.org).
- Download and review temperatures at least weekly.
- Keep the temperature data for at least 3 years.

Additional Best Practice Recommendations for Vaccine Storage and Handling[1,2]

- Designate a pharmacy staff person to oversee the storage and handling of vaccines.
- Identify a second person who will oversee vaccine storage and handling in the event the designated individual is unavailable.
- Be familiar with all storage and handling guidelines pertaining to the equipment and vaccines used.
- Develop written policies for routine and emergency vaccine storage and handling; review them with staff upon hiring and annually thereafter.
- Maintain a vaccine inventory log that contains the following:
  - Vaccine name
  - Number of doses received
  - Date of receipt

continued on page 40

Additional Best Practice Recommendations for Vaccine Storage and Handling, *continued from page 39*

  - o Condition of vaccine upon arrival
  - o Vaccine manufacturer and lot number
  - o Vaccine expiration date
- As new shipments are received, rotate the vaccine supply so that the items with the longest expiration dates are placed at the back.
- Routinely check vaccine expiration dates, and use the vaccines with the earliest expiration dates. Remember that expiration dates vary depending on vaccine or diluent type and lot number.
- Post a sign on the refrigerator that lists which vaccines should be kept refrigerated and which are frozen. This list should also highlight the appropriate storage of the respective diluents.

If a break in the cold chain occurs, it must be documented and steps must be taken to avoid use of the exposed vaccines until their potency and stability can be determined. If you suspect that the cold chain has been broken, separate the potentially damaged vaccines from the rest of the stock. Mark "Do Not Use" on the vials or unopened packaging. Continue to store these vaccines in the appropriate freezer or refrigerator compartments to preserve viability, in case you determine that you are able to use them. Contact your company's immunization or clinical coordinator, state health department, or vaccine manufacturer for additional guidance.

In addition to temperature sensitivity, many vaccines are sensitive to light. These vaccines, including manufacturer-filled syringes, should be stored in their original packaging, with the lids closed, at all times.[1] The specific storage conditions for commonly used vaccines can be found in Chapter 19 and in each vaccine's package insert. Vaccine manufacturers' recommendations and the vaccine storage and handling policies of your state health department should be followed. Contact your state health department and refer to the vaccine package insert for the most up-to-date information.

Prefilling or predrawing syringes prior to vaccine administration is not recommended.[1] The dose should be drawn up only when it is needed for immediate administration. The following problems may be introduced if syringes are prefilled:[1]

- Quality control can be compromised, since the person administering the vaccine may not be the one who filled the syringe.
- It is difficult to identify the vaccine in a prefilled syringe that is not properly labeled, and administration errors can result.
- Vaccine potency may be compromised; stability data are not available for vaccines stored in plastic syringes.
- Contamination is possible, especially if the vaccine does not contain preservatives or bacteriostatic agents.
- Vaccine will be wasted or stored improperly if more doses are pre-drawn than are needed.

Some exceptions have been made for mass immunization clinics; they are noted in Chapter 13.

Your vaccine inventory is expensive. Protecting your vaccine supply from improper storage conditions is critical. Both CDC and the Immunization Action Coalition (IAC) provide resources to help you and your staff manage the storage and handling of vaccines:

- CDC's Vaccine Storage and Handling Toolkit, available at www.cdc.gov/vaccines/recs/storage/toolkit/
- IAC's Clinic Resources for Storage and Handling, available at www.immunize.org/clinic/storage-handling.asp

References

1. Centers for Disease Control and Prevention. Vaccine Storage and Handling Toolkit. May 2014. www.cdc.gov/vaccines/recs/storage/toolkit/storage-handling-toolkit.pdf. Accessed September 28, 2014.
2. Immunization Action Coalition. Checklist for safe vaccine storage and handling. www.immunize.org/catg.d/p3035.pdf. Accessed September 28, 2014.

Figure 5.1
The Vaccine Cold Chain

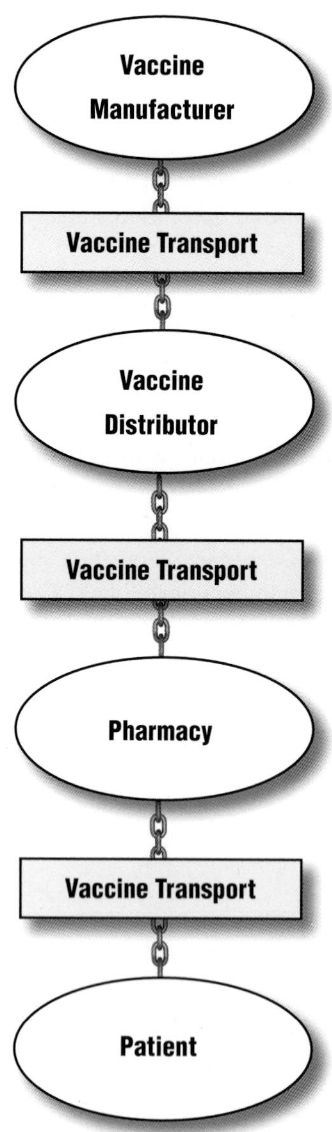

Adapted from: Reference 1.

Chapter 6

Creating Standing Orders and Protocols

A *standing order* is an order or directive for a specific action. In the context of pharmacists' provision of immunizations, it refers to a prescriptive order to administer a specific vaccine and is not limited to one particular patient. A *protocol* is the plan or process for carrying out a certain activity. In this case, it refers to the process for administration of vaccines or management of adverse reactions to vaccines. Both types of documents require preapproval and signature by a collaborating physician. Some physicians, and even state practice acts, may limit the number of patients to whom the standing order applies. Others may not have such a restriction, thereby granting permission to administer vaccines to an unlimited number of patients.

To improve vaccination rates among adults, adolescents, and children, the use of standing orders is encouraged.[1–3] Settings in which standing orders programs are recommended include inpatient, outpatient, assisted living, correctional, and long-term care facilities; managed care organizations; adult workplaces; home health care agencies; and pharmacies. The Centers for Medicare and Medicaid Services (CMS) highlights the use of standing orders programs as a best practice for improving the delivery of vaccinations.[4] CMS encourages the administration of vaccines by nurses and pharmacists using standing orders as an efficient means to provide seasonal influenza and pneumococcal mass immunizations.

If the pharmacy laws and regulations in your state allow you to administer vaccines pursuant to a standing order or protocol, then this chapter will be important to your immunization delivery service. If you are administering a vaccine pursuant to a standing order, you should have protocols in place that outline procedures for administration of the vaccine and for management of adverse reactions to the vaccine, including the use of epinephrine. If you will be administering multiple types of vaccines, then you should have a standing order for each vaccine.

Necessary Elements for Standing Orders and Protocols

The standing order and protocols for each vaccine to be administered should include the following:[1,5]

Vaccine administration

- Names and credentials of the individuals administering the vaccine
- Name of the practice site or location where the vaccine will be administered
- Effective dates of the standing order
- Name of vaccine to be administered
- Dose and route of the vaccine
- Criteria that must be met for a patient to receive the vaccine (e.g., age, risk factors, recurring dose in a series)
- Specified number of patients to whom the standing order applies, if applicable
- Screening process for contraindications and precautions
- Patient education to be provided, including delivery of the vaccine information statement (VIS)
- Documentation process
- Physician name, credentials, and signature
- Date signed

Medical management of adverse vaccine reactions

- Names and credentials of the individuals administering the vaccine
- Name of the practice site or location where the vaccine will be administered
- Effective dates of the protocol
- Reporting process to the Vaccine Adverse Event Reporting System (VAERS)
- Types of reactions possible, symptoms to expect, and management of such symptoms
  - Localized reaction
  - Syncope
  - Anaphylaxis
- Emergency management of anaphylactic reactions
  - Signs and symptoms to expect
  - Supplies needed to manage anaphylaxis

  - o Epinephrine dose and administration
  - o Diphenhydramine dose and administration, if applicable
  - o Notification of the emergency medical system (EMS)
  - o Monitoring process and use of cardiopulmonary resuscitation (CPR), if necessary
  - o Record keeping and physician follow-up
- Physician name, credentials, and signature
- Date signed

Examples of standing orders and administration protocols for specific vaccines, as well as the protocol for the medical management of vaccine reactions, are provided by the Immunization Action Coalition (IAC). These can be found on the IAC website at www.immunize.org/standing-orders and www.immunize.org/handouts/vaccine-reactions.asp, respectively.

A stepwise process for creating and implementing your standing order or protocols is as follows:

1. Determine whether you need a standing order, protocol, or both to administer vaccines in your state.
2. Determine which vaccine(s) you will be authorized to provide under a standing order or protocol, which also varies by state.
3. Determine which patients, on the basis of age, can be included on the standing order or protocol.
4. Draft the content, which should include the items noted previously.
5. Contact a local physician, preferably a primary care physician with whom you already have a relationship established, or a physician affiliated with your local health department.
6. Explain your service and reasons for collaboration to the physician.
7. Ask the physician to review the standing order or protocol.
8. Make any necessary changes subsequent to physician review.
9. Ask the physician to approve and sign the standing order or protocol.
10. Comply with any documentation and follow-up requirements the physician may have stipulated.

Standing Orders Programs for Inpatient Settings

In institutional settings or health-system environments, collaborative arrangements with physicians may already be established. In this instance, the physician, as well as other health care personnel integral to the vaccine delivery process, should be directly involved in creating the standing order or protocol with members of your pharmacy team. The use of a standing orders protocol, in which a pharmacist screened patients and activated a standing order to administer pneumococcal vaccinations to hospitalized patients, led to a 98% vaccination rate of eligible patients in the intervention ward in a 500-bed teaching hospital in New York.[6] The computerized reminder system used in a different ward in the same hospital resulted in only a 23% vaccination rate; this led to the use of a standing orders protocol on all general medicine wards at the hospital. Similarly, a tertiary care hospital in Pennsylvania reported vaccination rates of 15% in 2003, when a physician-reminder pneumococcal vaccination program was used.[7] The average rate increased to 69% in 2005, following the implementation of a standing orders program (SOP). Sokos et al.[7] noted that the low vaccination rates with the physician-reminder system were due to unsigned orders, lack of specific instructions on the order, and lack of knowledge about immunizations. Such barriers were considered in developing the SOP. The steps in implementing the SOP were as follows:[7]

1. Create the standing order form.
2. Incorporate vaccine documentation into the medication administration record (MAR).
3. Develop a vaccine kit to be sent from the pharmacy with each vaccine order. The kit contains the vaccine, MAR documentation forms or stickers (when electronic records are not used), the VIS, and a wallet card for the patient.
4. Determine who will maintain the SOP (e.g., pharmacy or nursing staff).
5. Design the flow of the SOP and define the roles of pharmacy personnel and nursing staff (Figure 6.1).
6. Develop a written hospital policy, which includes the intent of the standing order, defined roles, documentation process, and follow-up with primary care physicians.
7. Design and deliver educational programming to physicians, nursing staff and administration, unit clerks, and pharmacy personnel. Use immunization champions from each department to deliver educational messages.
8. Continuously assess SOP quality (e.g., monitor vaccination rates and omitted doses).

References

1. Advisory Committee on Immunization Practices. Use of standing orders programs to increase adult vaccination rates. *MMWR Recomm Rep.* 2000;49(RR-1):15–26. www.cdc.gov/mmwr/preview/mmwrhtml/rr4901a2.htm. Accessed October 5, 2014.
2. Elam-Evans LD, Yankey D, Jeyarajah J, et al. National, regional, state, and selected local area vaccination coverage among adolescents aged 13–17 years—United States, 2013. *MMWR Morb Mortal Wkly Rep.* 2014;63(29):625–33.
3. Community Preventive Services Task Force. Increasing appropriate vaccination: standing orders. www.thecommunityguide.org/vaccines/standingorders.html. Accessed October 5, 2014.
4. Centers for Medicare and Medicaid Services. Adult Immunization Resources for Providers. www.cms.gov/Medicare/Prevention/Immunizations/Providerresources.html. Accessed October 5, 2014.
5. Immunization Action Coalition. Standing orders for administering influenza vaccine to adults. www.immunize.org/catg.d/p3074.pdf. Accessed October 5, 2014.
6. Coyle CM, Currie BP. Improving the rates of inpatient pneumococcal vaccination: impact of standing orders versus computerized reminders to physicians. *Infect Control Hosp Epidemiol.* 2004;25:904–7.
7. Sokos DR, Skledar SJ, Ervin KA, et al. Designing and implementing a hospital-based vaccine standing orders program. *Am J Health Syst Pharm.* 2007;64:1096–102.

Figure 6.1

Example Flow of an Inpatient Standing Orders Program

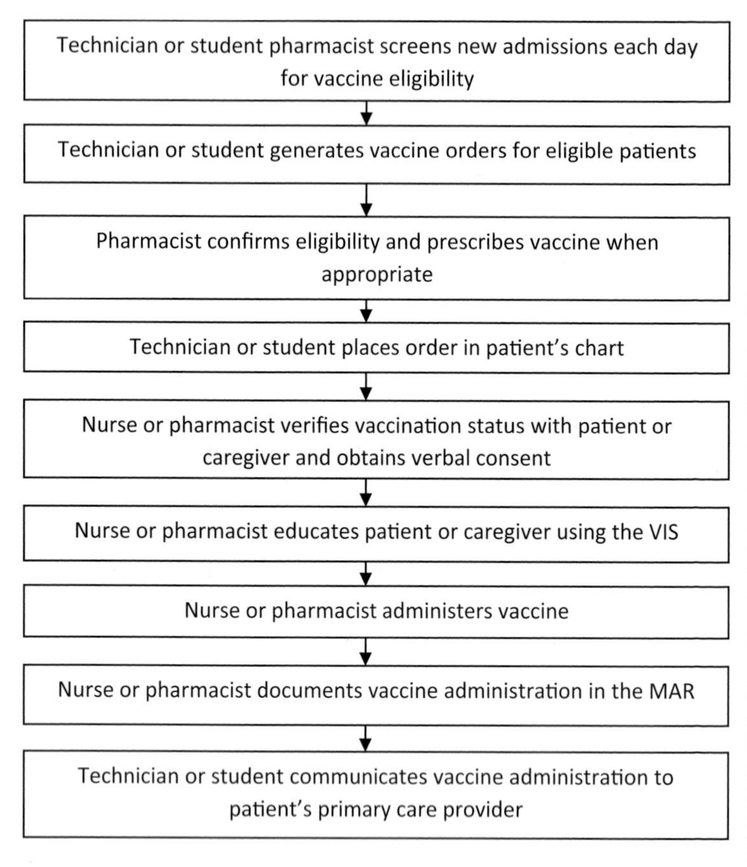

Adapted from: Reference 7.

Chapter 7

Billing for the Vaccine Product and Administration

Getting paid for the vaccine-delivery service you provide can be a daunting and cumbersome task, but it is an important one if this is to be a sustainable service. The National Vaccine Advisory Committee (NVAC) notes several barriers to adult vaccination in the 2014 Standards for Adult Immunization Practices report; most of these involve payment and coverage issues.[1] Provider recognition by third-party payers, use of only in-network providers, Medicare coverage limits, and Medicaid coverage variations by state are examples of barriers highlighted in the report. To overcome some of these reimbursement and compensation challenges, it will be helpful to determine what billing information you need and create a standardized billing process.

Many payers reimburse for vaccines. The extent to which you interact with them will depend on your geographic area and patient demographics. Table 7.1 lists most of the resources and forms you will need to use in billing for vaccines and vaccine administration. Before you begin billing, regardless of the payer type, you or your pharmacy will need to obtain a National Provider Identifier (NPI).

> Even if your pharmacy or employer has a National Provider Identifier (NPI), as a health care provider you should get one, too. It is simple to obtain and free of charge. The more pharmacists that obtain provider numbers, the stronger will be the argument that pharmacists are important providers of health care and should be recognized as such.

Medicare Part B

Your patients who are enrolled in Medicare Part B are eligible to receive the seasonal influenza and pneumococcal vaccines. Medicare will pay for one seasonal influenza immunization each year. Coverage of pneumococcal immunization is based on age and risk factors.[2,3] High-risk beneficiaries are eligible for a second pneumococcal immunization if 5 years have passed since they were last vaccinated. As of September 19, 2014, Medicare covers both the pneumococcal conjugate and polysaccharide vaccines for all adults 65 and older.[3] Long-term care facilities that participate in Medicare must offer annual influenza vaccination and pneumococcal immunization to eligible residents.[2] Pharmacists who consult for long-term care facilities should confirm that these vaccination requirements have been met during medication reviews. The hepatitis B vaccine is also covered by Medicare Part B for some beneficiaries considered to be at intermediate to high risk for the hepatitis B virus (HBV). Examples include health care workers who routinely work with blood or other potentially infectious materials, those with end-stage renal disease, those who reside with HBV-infected persons, and those with diabetes.[4] Other vaccines may be covered if they are indicated as a result of an injury or exposure to disease. A Part B beneficiary does not need to meet his or her deductible and is not responsible for a copayment for the influenza and pneumococcal vaccines. The deductible and copayment are required for the hepatitis B vaccine.[2]

As an individual pharmacist, you can apply to be a Medicare provider. However, if you work for a company that employs other pharmacists, then the pharmacy will likely be considered the provider and will be assigned the appropriate identifiers and numbers. A pharmacy or individual pharmacist can either enroll online via the Internet-based Provider Enrollment, Chain and Ownership System (PECOS) or fill out a paper application. If a paper application is completed, it will need to be mailed to the Medicare fee-for-service contractor (i.e., local carrier) for your state. The process for pharmacist and pharmacy enrollment is essentially the same. However, the forms and required information differ. The Centers for Medicare and Medicaid Services (CMS) requires individuals to complete form CMS-855I and pharmacies to complete form CMS-855B. If you are enrolling as a new Medicare provider, you will also need to complete form CMS-588, which will allow you to receive payment via electronic funds transfer. As of March 25, 2011, an application fee has been imposed, which may vary from year to year.[5] It can take up to 2 months to receive your provider number.[6,7] When preparing to provide your vaccine service, you will need to account for this time interval.

To enroll online, you must establish a National Plan and Provider Enumeration System (NPPES) Web user account; this is done when you apply for your NPI number. The NPPES user identification number and password are used to access the Internet-based PECOS.

If you have enrollment questions, contact your local Medicare carrier (see Table 7.1).

Billing Medicare Part B

You can bill Medicare for each beneficiary separately, or you can submit a roster bill. Billing can be done either electronically or using paper claims. Electronic submissions are preferred, since they are more efficient and environmentally friendly; however, some local carriers may not offer electronic roster billing.[8] Contact your local carrier to determine what billing methods exist.

Billing for both the vaccine product and administration is done via the CMS-1500 form, which is the Health Insurance Claim Form. If you administer more than one type of vaccine to a Medicare beneficiary, then each product must be listed on a separate line, with its respective administration code on the next line.[4] The diagnosis and administration codes are listed in Table 7.2.[4,8] The vaccine product codes (CPT® and HCPCS codes) are specific to each vaccine product. These codes should be looked up when they are needed for billing purposes. They are listed in Chapter 19 and can also be obtained from the following:

- Vaccine manufacturers
- Centers for Medicare and Medicaid Services—Quick Reference Information (www.cms.gov/Outreach-and-Education/Medicare-Learning-Network-MLN/MLNProducts/downloads/qr_immun_bill.pdf)
- Centers for Medicare and Medicaid Services—Immunizer's Guide (www.cms.gov/Medicare/Prevention/Immunizations/Downloads/2012-2013_Flu_Guide.pdf)

- Centers for Medicare and Medicaid Services—CPT Codes Mapped to CVX Codes (www2a.cdc.gov/vaccines/iis/iisstandards/vaccines.asp?rpt=cpt)

If both the influenza and the pneumococcal vaccines are administered during the same visit, use diagnosis code V06.6 along with the respective vaccine and administration codes. The patient needs to sign and date the form, or you can note "signature on file." If you do the latter, you must have a documented patient signature on file in your pharmacy. An auditor will look for such paperwork.

Roster bills are used for mass vaccination programs and must include at least two patients per form submission.[8] Roster billing can be done only for pneumococcal and influenza vaccines. You can use CMS-1500 forms that you have preprinted with the information listed in Table 7.3; however, each vaccine type must be billed on a separate form.[8] If you are a pharmacist who roster bills, your local carrier will likely prefer that you enroll individually using form CMS-855I. This will allow you to provide vaccinations off-site, so long as your address noted is the location at which your records are stored.[9] If you are enrolled with Medicare as a mass immunizer who roster bills, you must accept assignment as payment in full; you cannot bill the beneficiary for additional fees or costs. In addition, you will not be able to bill Medicare for any services other than influenza and pneumococcal vaccinations unless you change your specialty type. Along with the preprinted CMS-1500 form, you must submit a roster or log containing the following information for each patient:[8]

- Patient's health insurance claim number
- Patient's name and address
- Patient's date of birth
- Patient's sex
- Date of vaccine administration
- Vaccine administrator's name, NPI, and Medicare number (this will be either your number or your pharmacy's number)
- Patient's signature or "signature on file" notation

A roster bill template has been developed by the Immunization Action Coalition. It can be found in Appendix A of "Adults Only Vaccination:

A Step-by-Step Guide," located at www.immunize.org/guide/aovguide_all.pdf.

Medicare Part D

Medicare Part D, the prescription drug benefit for Medicare beneficiaries, covers those vaccines that are not covered by Part B (e.g., herpes zoster virus vaccine and Tdap). The prescription drug plans (PDPs) are required to cover vaccines that are reasonably necessary for the prevention of illness.[10] The negotiated price for the vaccine includes both product and administration.[10] CMS prefers that both vaccine product and administration be billed on one claim to avoid inadvertent duplicate billing of the administration fee, which could be considered a fraud and abuse violation.

In January 2008, use of the National Council for Prescription Drug Programs (NCPDP) telecommunications standard version 5.1 became required for billing Part D for the vaccine and its administration fee.[11] This requirement presented problems for physicians who wished to provide Part D covered vaccines to their patients. Patients often had to pay their physicians out-of-pocket for the vaccine and submit a claim to their PDPs for reimbursement. CMS has encouraged PDPs to develop electronic billing integration with physicians' offices to allow physicians to more efficiently bill for vaccines.[10] A letter written on behalf of 23 professional medical associations to the Department of Health and Human Services recognizes this billing issue and has suggested that Medicare Part B cover all preventive vaccines.[12]

You must have a contract with the patient's PDP in order to be reimbursed. As of January 1, 2012, all entities covered by the Health Insurance Portability and Accountability Act of 1996 (HIPAA) were required to be compliant with NCPDP version D.0.[13] Vaccine billing requirements for Part D should remain the same as in version 5.1 of the standard.[14] Certain pricing and DUR/PPS segments will need to be filled in when you are billing for vaccine product and administration (Table 7.4).[15] The Reason for Service Code (439-E4) and Result of Service Code (441-E6) fields are generally considered optional. If the vaccine product is dispensed but not administered, these administration codes should not be used. In addition, most claims will be denied if only the administration claim is submitted; the dispensing fee must be submitted in the same transaction. As updated NCPDP telecommunications standards are released, submission requirements and coding may change. Refer to the specific PDPs' payer sheets and work with the PDPs to determine the submission process for vaccine billing.

Medicaid, CHIP, and VFC

The Children's Health Insurance Program (CHIP), established in 1997, provides federal funding to states for insurance coverage for uninsured children.[16] Immunizations are included under CHIP, and Medicaid may be one of the avenues states use to provide this coverage. Each state Medicaid program determines its own eligibility requirements. Contact your state Medicaid program for more information on vaccine coverage for patients eligible for Medicaid. Visit www.insurekidsnow.gov for CHIP and Medicaid program-specific information in your state.

The Vaccines for Children (VFC) program, established in 1993, is the likely source of funding for vaccines for children who cannot afford them and whose insurance plans do not cover them. VFC provides vaccines at no cost to the recipient via grant-funded affiliations with the CDC. Children 18 years of age or younger who are eligible for Medicaid, as well as uninsured, underinsured, and American Indian or Alaska Native children, qualify for VFC-covered vaccines. If, however, the child is enrolled separately in the state's CHIP, he or she is not entitled to VFC program benefits.[17] For information on becoming a VFC program provider, contact your state's program coordinator. Visit www.cdc.gov/vaccines/programs/vfc/index.html for more information about VFC programs.

TRICARE Pharmacy Benefit

The TRICARE program provides health care benefits to active and retired members of the uniformed services and their dependents. In July 2011, the pharmacy benefit for TRICARE was expanded to include immunizations, allowing retail network pharmacies to administer vaccines.[18] The vaccines covered are those that are considered preventive and routinely recommended by CDC, including travel vaccines so long as the travel is performed pursuant to orders issued by the uniformed service. The Department of Defense (DoD) anticipates that costs will be saved by shifting immunizations from the medical to the pharmacy benefit.

Eligible TRICARE beneficiaries should not be charged a copayment for immunizations received at network pharmacies.

The Affordable Care Act and Other Payers

The Affordable Care Act has expanded coverage for vaccine-preventable diseases. Any new health insurance plan or policy beginning on or after September 23, 2010, must cover immunizations recommended by ACIP without charging a deductible, copayment, or coinsurance.[19] There are two caveats, however. First, this applies only if the vaccines are administered by an in-network provider. Second, if a new ACIP recommendation is made, coverage requirements take effect in the plan year that occurs one year after the effective recommendation date.

If you are unsure about immunization coverage for a patient, you can either contact the plan administrator directly for vaccine coverage information or attempt to submit the claim for the vaccine and adjudicate the claim according to the submission response. Do not prepare or administer the vaccine until coverage is determined and communicated to the patient. Electronic billing will likely be similar to other prescription-processing procedures, but be sure that vaccine administration is also included. If a claim is denied, the beneficiary can attempt to submit a universal claim form to the payer for reimbursement. If vaccine administration is not covered by the plan, you will need to bill the patient for this separately.

The billing codes and fields will likely be the same as those outlined for Medicare Part D claims. The current procedural terminology (CPT®) codes for commonly administered vaccines can be found with the product information in Chapter 19 and are listed on the CDC website (see Table 7.1). The diagnostic codes from the International Classification of Diseases, 9th Revision, Clinical Modification (ICD-9-CM), which often accompany the CPT® codes in billing for vaccines, are available through the CMS website (see Table 7.1). Note that the ICD-10 code set is expected to replace ICD-9 codes on October 1, 2015.[20] If diagnostic codes are required for reimbursement, specific codes must be used depending on the encounter and the vaccine administered.[21]

Local employer groups and regional health insurance providers may also be willing to cover vaccines for their employees or beneficiaries. If such opportunities exist in your area, take full advantage of them. This would be an excellent means to partner with a payer, expand your immunization service, and meet the vaccine needs of patients in your community.

Vaccine billing tips

- Obtain a National Provider Identifier for both you and your pharmacy.
- Obtain a Medicare provider number for either you or your pharmacy.
- Determine which payment method your patient is planning to use (i.e., Medicaid, Medicare Part B or D, another third-party plan, or self-pay).
- Assign the task of billing for vaccines and adjudicating claims to select individuals.
- Complete the respective billing forms, either electronically or on paper.
- Bill for both product reimbursement and administration compensation.
- Follow up to ensure that appropriate payment is received in a timely fashion.

References

1. National Vaccine Advisory Committee. Recommendations from the National Vaccine Advisory Committee: Standards for Adult Immunization Practices. *Public Health Rep.* 2014;129:115–23. www.publichealthreports.org/issueopen.cfm?articleID=3145. Accessed October 5, 2014.

2. Centers for Medicare and Medicaid Services. Adult immunization resources for providers. www.cms.gov/Medicare/Prevention/Immunizations/Providerresources.html. Accessed October 5, 2014.

3. Centers for Medicare and Medicaid Services. Modifications to Medicare Part B coverage of pneumococcal vaccinations. www.cms.gov/outreach-and-education/Medicare-learning-network-MLN/MLNMattersarticles/downloads/MM9051.pdf. Accessed January 18, 2015.

4. Centers for Medicare and Medicaid Services. Medicare Learning Network. Quick Reference Information: Medicare Immunization Billing (Seasonal Influenza Virus, Pneumococcal, and Hepatitis B). www.cms.gov/Outreach-and-Education/Medicare-Learning-Network-MLN/MLNProducts/downloads/qr_immun_bill.pdf. Accessed October 5, 2014.

5. Centers for Medicare and Medicaid Services. Medicare application fee. www.cms.gov/Medicare/Provider-Enrollment-and-Certification/MedicareProviderSupEnroll/MedicareApplicationFee.html. Accessed October 5, 2014.

6. American Pharmacists Association. Pharmacy-Based Immunization Delivery: A National Certificate Program for Pharmacists. 11th ed. Washington, DC: American Pharmacists Association; 2009.

7. Ernst ME, Charlstrom CV, Currie JD, et al. Implementation of a community pharmacy-based influenza vaccination program. *J Am Pharm Assoc.* 1997;NS37:570–80.
8. Centers for Medicare and Medicaid Services. 2012–2013 immunizers' question & answer guide to Medicare Part B & Medicaid coverage of seasonal influenza and pneumococcal vaccinations. www.cms.gov/Medicare/Prevention/Immunizations/Downloads/2012-2013_Flu_Guide.pdf. Accessed October 5, 2014.
9. Centers for Medicare and Medicaid Services. Medicare program integrity manual. www.cms.gov/Regulations-and-Guidance/Guidance/Transmittals/downloads/R29PIM.pdf. Accessed October 5, 2014.
10. Centers for Medicare and Medicaid Services. Reimbursement for vaccines and vaccine administration under Medicare Part D. MLN Matters SE0727. www.cms.gov/Outreach-and-Education/Medicare-Learning-Network-MLN/MLNMattersArticles/downloads/SE0727.pdf. Accessed October 5, 2014.
11. Centers for Medicare and Medicaid Services. Memorandum by Cynthia Tudor, 14 May 2007. Vaccine administration. www.cms.hhs.gov/PrescriptionDrugCovContra/Downloads/MemoVaccineAdministration_05.14.07.pdf. Accessed July 11, 2011.
12. Infectious Diseases Society of America. IDSA reaffirms its support of a Part D to Part B shift for all Medicare-covered vaccines (June 25, 2009). http://idsociety.org/View_All_Letters_on_Access_and_Reimbursement/. Accessed November 15, 2011.
13. Centers for Medicare and Medicaid Services. Electronic billing and EDI transactions. 5010 – D.0. www.cms.gov/Medicare/Billing/ElectronicBillingEDITrans/18_5010D0.html. Accessed October 5, 2014.
14. National Council for Prescription Drug Programs. NCPDP payer sheet template: implementation guide for version D.0. Version 1.4. August 2011.
15. National Council for Prescription Drug Programs. Telecommunication version 5 questions, answers and editorial updates (November 2010). www.ncpdp.org/members/pdf/Version5.Editorial.pdf. Accessed October 5, 2014.
16. Centers for Medicare and Medicaid Services. Letter to State Health Officials (May 11, 1998). www.cms.hhs.gov/smdl/downloads/sho051198.pdf. Accessed October 5, 2014.
17. Centers for Medicare and Medicaid Services. VFC: eligibility criteria. www.cdc.gov/vaccines/programs/vfc/providers/eligibility.html. Accessed October 5, 2014.
18. U.S. Department of Defense. Civilian Health and Medical Program of the Uniformed Services (CHAMPUS)/TRICARE: Inclusion of retail network pharmacies as authorized TRICARE providers of TRICARE covered vaccines, final rule. *Federal Register.* 2011(Jul 13);76(134):41063.

19. U.S. Department of Health & Human Services. The Affordable Care Act and Immunization. www.hhs.gov/healthcare/facts/factsheets/2010/07/preventive-services-list.html. Accessed October 5, 2014.
20. American Medical Association. ICD-10 Code Set to Replace IDC-9. www.ama-assn.org/ama/pub/physician-resources/solutions-managing-your-practice/coding-billing-insurance/hipaahealth-insurance-portability-accountability-act/transaction-code-set-standards/icd10-code-set.page. Accessed October 5, 2014.
21. American Academy of Pediatrics. Coding for vaccines and immunization administration in 2011: major and welcome changes to the *CPT* 2011 immunization administration codes. *AAP Pediatric Coding Newsletter Online.* November 2010. http://coding.aap.org/content.aspx?aid=11390. Accessed July 8, 2011.

Table 7.1

Internet Resources and Forms for Billing

National Plan and Provider Enumeration System (NPPES): National Provider Identifier (NPI) application	https://nppes.cms.hhs.gov/NPPES/Welcome.do
CMS-1500 form (sample)	www.cms.gov/Medicare/CMS-Forms/CMS-Forms/downloads/CMS1500805.pdf
CMS-855B enrollment application	www.cms.gov/Medicare/CMS-Forms/CMS-Forms/downloads/cms855b.pdf
CMS-855I enrollment application	www.cms.gov/Medicare/CMS-Forms/CMS-Forms/downloads/cms855i.pdf
CMS-588 form (Electronic Funds Transfer Authorization Agreement)	www.cms.gov/Medicare/CMS-Forms/CMS-Forms/downloads/CMS588.pdf
CMS adult immunization resources for providers	www.cms.gov/Medicare/Prevention/Immunizations/index.html
Medicare provider/supplier enrollment resources	www.cms.gov/Medicare/Provider-Enrollment-and-Certification/MedicareProviderSupEnroll/index.html

continued on page 59

Local Medicare carrier contact list (by state)	www.cms.gov/Medicare/Provider-Enrollment-and-Certification/MedicareProviderSupEnroll/downloads/contact_list.pdf
State contacts for health insurance for children	www.insurekidsnow.gov/state/index.html
State Vaccines for Children contact information	www.cdc.gov/vaccines/programs/vfc/contacts-state.html
CDC vaccine price list	www.cdc.gov/vaccines/programs/vfc/awardees/vaccine-management/price-list/index.html
Vaccine CPT® codes	www2a.cdc.gov/vaccines/IIS/IISStandards/vaccines.asp?rpt=cpt
ICD-9-CM and ICD-10 provider and diagnostic code resources	www.cms.gov/Medicare/Coding/ICD9ProviderDiagnosticCodes/index.html

CMS = Centers for Medicare and Medicaid Services.

Table 7.2

Seasonal Influenza, Pneumococcal, and Hepatitis B Vaccine Diagnosis and Administration Codes

Vaccine	Diagnosis Code (Item 21)[a]	Administration Code (Item 24D)[a]
Seasonal influenza virus vaccine	V04.81	G0008
Pneumococcal vaccine	V03.82	G0009
Hepatitis B vaccine	V05.3	G0010

[a]Item numbers in column headings refer to areas of the CMS-1500 claim form.
Adapted from: References 4 and 8.

Table 7.3

Information to Preprint on CMS-1500 Claim Form for Influenza and Pneumococcal Vaccines Roster Billing

Item	Information to Include
1	"X" in the MEDICARE box
2	"See attached roster" for PATIENT'S NAME
11	"None" for INSURED'S POLICY GROUP OR FECA NUMBER
20	"X" in the NO box for OUTSIDE LAB?
21	Insert respective diagnosis code (see Table 7.2)
24B	"60" for PLACE OF SERVICE in both Lines 1 and 2
24D, Line 1[a]	Insert respective CPT® code (see Chapter 18)
24D, Line 2	Insert respective administration code (see Table 7.2)
24E	"1" for DIAGNOSIS POINTER in both Lines 1 and 2
24F	Enter the charge for the vaccine
27	"Yes" for ACCEPT ASSIGNMENT?
29	"$0.00" for AMOUNT PAID
31	Sign and date the form
32	Enter the name, address, and ZIP code for the location where the vaccines were provided
32a	Enter the NPI of the facility or pharmacy where the vaccines were provided
33	Enter your name and phone number
33a	Enter your NPI

[a] *Confirm that the CPT code entered for item 24D, Line 1 corresponds with the specific vaccine product used.*

Adapted from: Reference 8.

Table 7.4

Select Fields to Populate When Billing for Vaccines Using NCPDP vD.0

Segment	Field Number	Field Name	Value
Claim	455-EM	Prescription/Service Reference Number Qualifier	"1" (Default value since value does not exist for product/service combination)
Pricing	409-D9*	Ingredient Cost Submitted	Vaccine product cost
Pricing	412-DC*	Dispensing Fee Submitted	Dispensing fee
Pricing	438-E3	Incentive Amount (or Fee) Submitted	Vaccine administration fee
Pricing	426-DQ*	Usual and Customary Charge	Vaccine drug cost + administration fee that would be charged to patient (sum of 409-D9, 412-DC, and 438-E3)
Pricing	430-DU*	Gross Amount Due	Summation of ingredient cost, dispensing fee, and incentive fee
DUR/PPS	473-7E	DUR/PPS Code Counter	"1" (indicates claim is being submitted for vaccine administration)
DUR/PPS	440-E5	Professional Service Code	"MA" (medication administration)

NCPDP = National Council for Prescription Drug Programs.

**May be optional depending on plan; refer to respective payer sheet for required fields.*

Source: Reference 15.

Chapter 8

Record Keeping and Documentation

Immunization Records

It is recommended that immunization records be kept for a patient's lifetime. However, what is actually required by law varies by state and is often consistent with the pharmacy's other prescription record-keeping requirements. The Centers for Medicare and Medicaid Services (CMS) mandates retention times for Medicare Part D prescription records and Medicare Part B claims. Part D prescription records must be kept for at least 10 years; they must be kept in their original format for 3 years and can be transferred to electronic format for the remaining 7 years.[1,2] Medicare Part B claims records must be kept for 6 years and 3 months following the close of the calendar year in which the claim is paid; if converted to microfilm, the original claims records can be destroyed after 3 years following the close of the calendar year in which the claim is paid.[3,4] Check your state's laws and regulations to determine how long you must keep your patients' immunization records, as a state's requirements may be more stringent than the federal requirements. Regardless of these requirements, always encourage your patients to keep their own immunization records current and in a readily accessible location. Offer to update their records each time vaccines are administered.

Vaccine Administration Documentation

Federal law requires that vaccine administrators document the following information in the patient's permanent medical record:[5]

- Date of vaccine administration
- Vaccine manufacturer
- Vaccine lot number
- Name, address, and title of the health care provider administering the vaccine
- The edition date of the vaccine information statement (VIS)
- Date the VIS was provided

The National Childhood Vaccine Injury Act of 1986 (42 U.S.C. Sec. 300aa-26) mandates this documentation only for the following vaccines, or combinations thereof:[5]

- Diphtheria, tetanus, pertussis (DTP, DTaP, Tdap, DT, Td, or TT)
- *Haemophilus influenzae* type b (Hib)
- Hepatitis A (HAV)
- Hepatitis B (HBV)
- Human papillomavirus (HPV)
- Influenza (TIV, LAIV)
- Measles, mumps, rubella (MMR, MR, M, R)
- Meningococcal (MCV, MPSV)
- Polio
- Pneumococcal conjugate
- Rotavirus
- Varicella

However, it is recommended that you apply the aforementioned documentation requirements to all vaccines you administer.

Consent Forms

Although there is no federal law requiring patient or caregiver informed consent for immunizations, your state law or company policy may require the use of consent forms. Most states require parental or legal representative consent for vaccines to be administered to children or adolescents.[6,7]

Vaccination Information for Physicians

As a pharmacist providing immunizations, it is your responsibility to notify your patient's primary care physician that the vaccination was administered.[8] This reporting may also be required by your state law. Depending on the agreed-upon terms of the standing order or protocol, you may be expected to send this information to the collaborating physician as well. Such communication with physicians not only serves to maintain the patient's immunization status in his or her permanent medical record at the physician's office, but it also helps to increase physicians' awareness and appreciation of the service and collaborative arrangement.[8,9] The information sent to the physician should include, at a minimum, the following:[8,9]

- Patient's name
- Patient's date of birth
- Patient's identification or medical record number (if known)
- Administering pharmacist's name and contact information
- Name of vaccine and dose administered
- Site of injection
- Date of vaccine administration
- Vaccine manufacturer and lot number

This information can be communicated in a variety of ways; facsimile (fax) transmission and U.S. mail are probably the most common. A template or form should be created to keep the type and extent of communication consistent from one patient to the next. If numerous patients see the same physician, you may be able to send this information in bulk in the form of a roster or log at agreed-upon intervals. You will need to create and maintain a database or spreadsheet to track this type of information. If deemed beneficial by the physician or office staff, who may still be using paper charts, you can provide chart stickers to simplify the process of updating the patient's medical record.

Immunization Information Systems

Immunization information systems (IIS), otherwise known as immunization registries, offer a confidential, computerized means of capturing population-based vaccination data for a specific geographic area.[10] The use of these systems or registries has been shown to increase immunization rates and reduce vaccine-preventable diseases by facilitating timely interventions, assisting in vaccination status assessment, guiding the response to outbreaks, identifying coverage gaps, and facilitating vaccine management and accountability.[11] The systems are managed at the state level, but data are tracked separately for some major U.S. cities.[12] According to data for 2013, New Hampshire was the only state that did not have an IIS.[12] Initially, these systems were developed to track the immunization status of each child to allow multiple providers convenient and timely access to the data, but many of them have been expanded to include adolescents and adults. In fact, two of the Healthy People 2020 objectives are to have at least 95% IIS participation of children less than 6 years of age and to increase to at least 40 the number of states with 80% participation for adolescents age 11 to 18.[13] According to CDC's 2013 IIS Annual Report, national participation was 90% for children less than 6 years of age and 64% for adolescents.[12] Many states mandate IIS reporting, especially for children. Check with your state to determine whether these reporting laws apply to your practice.

If you are involved in childhood immunization or want to learn more about the IIS reporting options in your state, contact your state's registry staff. The contact information can be found at www.cdc.gov/vaccines/programs/iis/contacts-registry-staff.html.

OSHA Record-Keeping Requirements

As detailed in Chapter 17, certain employee records must be maintained under the Occupational Safety and Health Administration (OSHA) Bloodborne Pathogens Standard (Table 8.1).[14] A workbook and forms for recording work-related injuries can be found on the OSHA website.[15]

References

1. Centers for Medicare and Medicaid Services. Medicare prescription drug benefit: solicitation for applications for new prescription drug plan (PDP) sponsors, 2012 contract year. www.cms.gov/PrescriptionDrugCovContra/Downloads/PDPApplication.pdf. Accessed October 7, 2014.
2. Contract provisions. 42 CFR §423.505 (2010).
3. Limitations. 42 CFR §1003.132 (2009).
4. Centers for Medicare and Medicaid Services. Centers for Medicare and Medicaid Services (CMS) records schedule. September 2014. www.cms.gov/Regulations-and-Guidance/Guidance/CMSRecordsSchedule/Downloads/RecordsSchedule.pdf. Accessed October 7, 2014.
5. Centers for Disease Control and Prevention. Instructions for using VISs. www.cdc.gov/vaccines/hcp/vis/about/required-use-instructions.html. Accessed October 7, 2014.
6. Gordon TE, Zook EG, Averhoff FM, et al. Consent for adolescent vaccination: issues and current practices [abstract]. *J Sch Health.* 1997;67(7).
7. Ernst ME, Chalstrom CV, Currie JD, et al. Implementation of a community pharmacy-based influenza vaccination program. *J Am Pharm Assoc.* 1997;NS37:570–80.

8. English A, Shaw FE, McCauley MM, et al. Legal basis of consent for health care and vaccination for adolescents. *Pediatrics.* 2008;121(Suppl 1):S85–7. doi:10.1542/10.1542/peds.2007-1115J.

9. Weitzel KW, Goode JR. Implementation of a pharmacy-based immunization program in a supermarket chain. *J Am Pharm Assoc.* 2000;40:252–6.

10. Centers for Disease Control and Prevention. About Immunization Information Systems. www.cdc.gov/vaccines/programs/iis/about.html. Accessed October 7, 2014.

11. Community Preventive Services Task Force. Increasing Appropriate Vaccination: Immunization Information Systems. www.thecommunityguide.org/vaccines/imminfosystems.html. Accessed October 7, 2014.

12. Centers for Disease Control and Prevention. Immunization Information Systems Annual Report (IISAR). www.cdc.gov/vaccines/programs/iis/annual-report-IISAR/index.html. Accessed October 7, 2014.

13. U.S. Department of Health and Human Services. 2020 topics and objectives: immunization and infectious diseases. www.healthypeople.gov/2020/topics-objectives/topic/immunization-and-infectious-diseases/objectives. Accessed October 7, 2014.

14. Bloodborne pathogens. 29 CFR §1910.1030 (2007). www.osha.gov/pls/oshaweb/owadisp.show_document?p_table=STANDARDS&p_id=10051. Accessed October 7, 2014.

15. U.S. Department of Labor, Occupational Safety and Health Administration. OSHA forms for recording work-related injuries and illnesses. www.osha.gov/recordkeeping/new-osha300form1-1-04.pdf. Accessed October 7, 2014.

Table 8.1

Record-Keeping Requirements under OSHA's Bloodborne Pathogens Standard

Type of Record	Time to Be Kept on File
Confidential medical record for employee with occupational exposure	Duration of employment plus 30 years
OSHA training record for each employee	3 years from the date of training
Sharps injury log	5 years following the year(s) in which incident(s) occurred

Source: Reference 14.

Chapter 9

Marketing Immunization Services

Once you have successfully laid the groundwork for offering immunizations, you will need to publicize the availability of this service. Your marketing efforts should be directed toward a variety of audiences, including patients, health care providers, community groups, media groups, employer groups, and your own employees. Each audience, however, will have different needs and expectations of the service, and effective marketing messages will reflect this (Table 9.1).[1,2]

To promote your influenza vaccination program, for example, you will find guidance and key communication points in a media relations toolkit routinely published by CDC. The toolkit, along with other promotional materials, is available at www.cdc.gov/flu/nivw/index.htm. Talking points provided by the CDC include the following:

- Influenza (the flu) is a serious disease that can lead to hospitalization and sometimes even death. Anyone can get sick from the flu.
- To date, most children who have died from the flu were not vaccinated against flu.
- Flu viruses are constantly changing. Each flu season, different flu viruses can spread, and they can affect people differently based on differences in the immune system. Even healthy children and adults can get very sick from the flu.
- A flu vaccination reduces your risk of illness, hospitalization, or even death.
- The flu vaccine is recommended for everyone 6 months of age and older, with rare exceptions.

If your immunization program includes pneumococcal vaccines, resources provided by the National Foundation for Infectious Diseases will be useful. Developed for health care providers who work with pneumococcal vaccines and educate patients on the disease, these resources include fact sheets, expert advice, a poster, newsletter and reminder email templates, and immunization assessment forms. The materials are available in English and Spanish and can be obtained at www.adultvaccination.org/professional-resources/practice-toolkit. Also included in this Professional Practice Toolkit are promotional resources for adult vaccinations (in general) that can be customized to your practice needs.

Whatever vaccination service or program you provide, it will be important to tailor your marketing activities and materials to emphasize the information most relevant to each audience.

Most marketing vehicles require significant investments of both time and financial resources. Depending on your practice site, you may already have certain resources available. For instance, if you work for a company or corporation, you may be able to combine your marketing efforts with those already under way for other events promoted by the organization. You may be able to collaborate with an internal marketing department. Or, marketing materials that have already been developed by the organization may be provided to you. If, however, you must single-handedly create your own marketing materials, Table 9.2 can be used to guide your marketing plan and development process.[3,4] Given the options and resources available, you can decide which combination of marketing vehicles will be best suited to your target audience. Keep in mind that any messages delivered directly to patients (e.g., telephone messages, mailings) should either be generic or use confidentiality measures to protect patient privacy.

Several recent studies have assessed the use of promotional strategies to increase herpes zoster vaccination rates. Some strategies shown to be effective are described below.

- A press release to newspapers, flyers distributed with prescriptions, and personalized letters were used during a 4-week intervention period.[5] All of these had a positive impact, but the personalized letter was the most effective.
- Signage and brochures were placed around two pharmacies; the study pharmacy also incorporated personal selling at the pharmacy, brochures attached to prescription bags, and personalized letters sent to half of the study group.[6] The study site had higher vaccination rates, and the personal selling and letters were described by patients as having a greater impact than the signs and brochure.

- Thirty-second prerecorded messages were delivered monthly by telephone for three months to an intervention group of 5599 patients. The result was a significantly higher vaccination rate than for the control group.[7]

A 2010 study of barriers to and facilitators of childhood immunization relied on focus groups consisting of health care professionals, parents, adolescents, and marketing professionals.[8] The groups' suggestions for marketing influenza vaccination to children and adolescents included office displays, cable television spots, items that can be worn, famous spokespersons, incentives, videos, jingles, and information sheets or posters. Regardless of the strategy used, the focus group members believed it was imperative that the information come from a trusted and informed source. As McDonough and colleagues[3] point out, your best promotional tool will be the quality of care that you provide to your patients. Information via word of mouth does not require a financial investment. Your investment, rather, is in the form of reputation and value. Satisfied patients and positive recognition from other health care providers can do wonders for your vaccine delivery service. Substandard care and poor quality will result in a negative image of your service. Continuous program evaluation and quality improvement initiatives are important in sustaining a profitable and well-regarded immunization practice.

Tips for developing print materials with a professional appearance

- Use a software program designed to help you create marketing materials (e.g., Microsoft Office templates, Microsoft Publisher, SmartDraw).
- Outsource design and printing of materials to a local company specializing in this service.
- Get the marketing text copyedited for punctuation, grammar, and spelling errors.
- Create text that is simple and easy for the consumer to read and understand, preferably at a grade 6 or lower reading level and free of complex medical terminology.
- Use an instrument or software program that assesses the health literacy level of documents (visit www.nlm.nih.gov/medlineplus/etr.html for readability assessment tools and programs).
- Avoid small and obscure fonts.
- Print in color.

Tips for audio advertisements and personal interviews

- Prepare relevant speaking points in advance.
- Repeatedly relay a consistent key message.
- Stick to the facts.
- Avoid verbal and nonverbal distracters (e.g., "um," "uh," "like," excessive hand or facial movements, poor posture, multicolored or patterned clothing).
- Speak clearly and eloquently.
- Avoid complex medical terminology.
- Request a verbal sound check.
- When interviewing in person, maintain eye contact.
- When speaking by telephone or on the radio, stand during the interview or the advertisement recording.
- Provide the audience with a simple and easy-to-recall way to obtain additional information.
- Prepare by reading a book or attending a seminar or workshop specializing in media and public relations training.
- Practice aloud, either in front of a video camera or with a voice recording device.

References

1. Harris IM, Baker E, Berry TM, et al. Developing a business-practice model for pharmacy services in ambulatory settings. *Pharmacotherapy.* 2008;28:285. www.accp.com/docs/positions/whitePapers/AmbCareBusPractModelACCP.pdf. Accessed October 8, 2014.

2. Snella KA, Sachdev GP. A primer for developing pharmacist-managed clinics in the outpatient setting. *Pharmacotherapy.* 2003;23:1153–66.

3. McDonough RP, Pithan ES, Doucette WR, et al. Marketing pharmaceutical care services. *J Am Pharm Assoc.* 1998;38:667–81.

4. Weitzel KW, Goode JR. Implementation of a pharmacy-based immunization program in a supermarket chain. *J Am Pharm Assoc.* 2000;40:252–6.

5. Wang J, Ford LJ, Wingate L, et al. The effect of pharmacist intervention on herpes zoster vaccination in community pharmacies. *J Am Pharm Assoc.* 2013;53(1):46–53.

6. Bryan AR, Liu Y, Kuehl PG. Advocating zoster vaccination in a community pharmacy through use of personal selling. *J Am Pharm Assoc.* 2013;53(1):70–9.

7. Hess R. Impact of automated telephone messaging on zoster vaccination rates in community pharmacies. *J Am Pharm Assoc.* 2013;53(2):182–7.

8. Bhat-Schelbert K, Lin CJ, Matambanadzo A, et al. Barriers to and facilitators of child influenza vaccine—perspectives from parents, teens, marketing and healthcare professionals. *Vaccine.* 2012;30(14):2448–52.

Additional Marketing Resources for Pharmacists

Holdford DA. *Marketing for Pharmacists.* 2nd ed. Washington, DC: American Pharmacists Association; 2007.
Pugliese TL. *Public Relations for Pharmacists.* 2nd ed. Washington, DC: American Pharmacists Association; 2008.

Table 9.1
Marketing Messages for Specific Audiences

Audience	Messages to Deliver
Patients	Reasons for being immunized against vaccine-preventable diseases, including vaccine safety and consequences of the disease Expected costs Time commitment to be vaccinated Process to follow to receive vaccines
Health care providers	Qualifications, training, and credentials of those providing immunizations Impact on patient morbidity and mortality Patient referral process Documentation and health care provider follow-up process
Community	Ability to offer the service at alternative locations (e.g., community group centers, senior citizen centers, churches, schools) Expected costs Scheduling and staffing process for immunization clinics
Media groups	Reasons patients should be immunized against vaccine-preventable diseases Impact of the service on the community Date, time, and location of the service

continued on page 74

Table 9.1

continued from page 73

Audience	Messages to Deliver
Employer groups	Cost savings of the immunization service Impact on employee morbidity and mortality (e.g., reduced sick days, reduced loss of productivity, reduced hospitalizations) Employee satisfaction with the service
Pharmacy personnel	Components of the immunization service Benefits of the service to communicate to patients Process patients need to follow to receive vaccines

Adapted from: References 1 and 2.

Table 9.2

Comparison of Marketing Tools

Marketing Vehicle	Financial Investment[a]	Time to Develop and Implement
Bag stuffers	$	🕘
Auxiliary labels	$	🕘
In-store signage	$$	🕘 🕘
Overhead announcements	$	🕘
Interactive voice response message	$	🕘
Promotional/educational pharmacy newsletter[3]	$	🕘 🕘 🕘
Social networking sites (e.g., Facebook, Twitter)	—	🕘
Opinion piece in local newspaper[3]	—	🕘 🕘
Press release for local media[3]	—	🕘 🕘
Community newsletter ad	$	🕘 🕘
Radio ad	$$$	🕘 🕘 🕘 🕘

continued on page 75

Local television ad	$$$	🕘 🕘 🕘 🕘 🕘
Newspaper ad	$$$	🕘 🕘
Weekly store circular ad	$$	🕘 🕘
Information posted on Flu Clinic Locator site	—	🕘
Vehicle magnets	—	🕘 🕘
Yellow Pages ad	$$$	🕘 🕘
Direct mailings	$$	🕘 🕘
Educational talks to community groups	$	🕘 🕘 🕘
Physician detailing and staff in-service	$	🕘 🕘 🕘
Chart stickers for physicians' offices[4]	$	🕘
Referral cards to be used by other pharmacies and health care providers	$	🕘 🕘
Patient education brochures	$	🕘 🕘
Promotion piece on company's website	$$	🕘 🕘 🕘
Word of mouth	—	—

[a]*Monetary requirements will vary depending on internal and organization resources already available.*

Chapter 10

Vaccine Reminder and Recall Systems

Many of the patients you vaccinate will need to receive another vaccine at some point in the future. This may be the influenza vaccine the following year or additional doses within a series. Encouraging patients to return to you to receive a recommended vaccine has several advantages:

- Helps to improve immunization rates[1]
- Maintains consistent and accurate immunization records
- Provides continuity of care
- Keeps patients healthy
- Sustains your immunization delivery service
- Complies with recommendations of the Advisory Committee on Immunization Practices and the Community Preventive Services Task Force regarding the use of reminder/recall systems[1,2]

The methods for reminders (for vaccines that are due) and recalls (for vaccines that are past due) should be tailored to both your patients and your pharmacy staff. If any of your messages to patients are personalized, remember to take precautions to protect patient privacy. The messages should come directly from you or your staff and be confidentially delivered to the patient or the patient's legal representative. For instance, if post cards are used in which the messaging can be seen by others, they should include generic vaccine awareness or marketing messages and should be addressed to the "Current Resident." If you are calling the patient and must leave a message with a recording machine or another person, do not include any health information about the patient; rather, simply ask that the patient return your call.

Reminder methods for patients and caregivers

- Telephone calls
- Letters
- Post cards
- Auxiliary labels
- Stamps or stickers on prescription bags
- Appointment cards distributed at initial visit
- Electronic mail
- Calendar reminders for hand-held electronic devices, input by patient at initial visit

Text messaging has been used to remind patients to receive influenza vaccines, but with varying degrees of effectiveness.[3–5] Advantages to using text messaging reminders are they can reach a large population of patients and provide simple and quickly accessible messages. However, technology must be in place to distribute text messages in bulk (through either external software vendors or internal immunization tracking systems/electronic health records with text messaging capability). This method also relies on having correct mobile phone numbers for patients, and the system must provide patients with the option to stop receiving texts.

For patient reminders to be generated at the appropriate times, a system will need to be in place to remind you and your staff to contact patients. Unfortunately, most computer systems used in pharmacies for prescription processing are not capable of tracking patient immunization status or generating reminders. In states with fully operational and up-to-date immunization information systems, these systems can be used to help identify patients in need of vaccines. Most likely, you will need to use a separate electronic program or resort to a paper tracking method. Here are some examples:

- Set up a Microsoft Excel spreadsheet with your patients' names, contact information, and dates of next scheduled vaccines. Sort the information by date.

- Create a program in Microsoft Access from which you can generate reminders and run reports of patients needing vaccines.
- Use an internal electronic calendar system to record when patients are due for their next vaccine.
- Place index cards with patients' names and contact information in a card file, organized by date of the next scheduled vaccine.
- Record patients' names and contact information in a planner or calendar.

If you choose to use your own hand-held electronic device to track reminders, be sure that the device is password protected. If it were lost or stolen, protected health and patient information could be breached or compromised. Regardless of the reminder system you select, someone will need to be assigned the task of routinely using the system to identify patients in need of their next scheduled vaccines. Follow-up will then be needed, using one of the messaging methods noted above. This is a great opportunity to involve technicians and student pharmacists in the immunization delivery service. Provide them with a scripted template to use when making phone calls or a letter template that can be generated using a mail merge function. A sample telephone script and letter can be found at www2a.cdc.gov/vaccines/ed/whatworks/pdfs/mailed_reminder.pdf. These will have to be redesigned to meet the needs of your practice site and to ensure that patient privacy is protected.

The major limitations in implementing successful reminder systems are time and resources. The ease of use and efficiency of your system will be key. Assigning specific pharmacy personnel to manage the reminders as a routine job function is also critical.

References

1. Centers for Disease Control and Prevention. *Epidemiology and Prevention of Vaccine-Preventable Diseases.* Atkinson W, Wolfe S, Hamborsky J, et al., eds. 12th ed. 2nd printing (May 2012). Washington, DC: Public Health Foundation; 2011.
2. Community Preventive Services Task Force. Increasing Appropriate Vaccination: Client Reminder and Recall Systems. www.thecommunityguide.org/vaccines/clientreminder.html. Accessed October 10, 2014.

3. Stockwell MS, Kharbanda EO, Martinez RA, et al. Effect of a text messaging intervention on influenza vaccination in an urban, low-income pediatric and adolescent population: a randomized controlled trial. *JAMA.* 2012;307(16):1702–8.
4. Stockwell MS, Westhoff C, Kharbanda EO, et al. Influenza vaccine text message reminders for urban, low-income pregnant women: a randomized controlled trial. *Am J Public Health.* 2014;104 Suppl 1:e7–12.
5. Moniz MH, Hasley S, Meyn LA, et al. Improving influenza vaccination rates in pregnancy through text messaging: a randomized controlled trial. *Obstet Gynecol.* 2013;121(4):734–40.

Chapter 11

Roles for Technicians and Student Pharmacists

Roles for Pharmacy Technicians

Just as technicians have an invaluable role in processing, filling, and dispensing medications in the pharmacy, they can be key players in the provision of immunization services. In fact, Goal 23 of the Model Curriculum for Pharmacy Technician Education and Training Programs states that technicians should be taught to "assist pharmacists in preparing, storing, and distributing medication products requiring special handling and documentation" and cites immunizations as one example.[1] Involving technicians in the immunization delivery service can help the pharmacy minimize interruptions in workflow, ensure safe and effective vaccine delivery, maintain appropriate documentation and record keeping, and efficiently process billing claims. Such support functions help to free up time for the pharmacist to administer vaccines.[2,3] In addition, encouraging technicians to participate in the immunization service can enhance their performance and job satisfaction. Even though the responsibilities of technicians have been expanded over the past several years, the feeling that they can contribute further to the practice site still remains.[4] Direct involvement in immunization services would be an excellent opportunity for increasing their job responsibilities. Technicians might perform the following activities:

- Process the vaccine prescription
- Update the patient's profile and immunization record
- Provide patients with the necessary screening forms to be completed for documentation purposes
- Distribute the appropriate vaccine information statements to patients
- Prepare the vaccine supplies
- Maintain pharmacy workflow and operations while the pharmacist is administering vaccines

- Fax any necessary communication to the patient's primary care provider
- Check and record daily temperatures for the refrigerator and freezer containing vaccines
- Check expiration dates of vaccines in stock
- Check expiration dates of epinephrine supply
- Maintain the vaccine supply and order vaccines when necessary
- Schedule appointments for patients to receive immunizations
- Call patients to remind them of their appointments
- Place vaccine reminder stickers on prescription vials and bags
- Promote the immunization service to patients and the community

To fulfill these tasks, technicians will need education and training. Not all technicians will be willing or able to take on the same degree of responsibility, and the activities in which they can be involved may be limited by your state's pharmacy laws and regulations. You will need to determine which activities can be appropriately delegated to your technicians and how to assign these activities on the basis of your assessment of the technician's ability to perform the tasks. The capabilities of individual technicians will determine the extent of training needed. Technicians' competence to assist in the immunization service will depend largely on the quality of training they receive. It may be advisable to consider two levels of training for technicians in your immunization service: basic and advanced (Table 11.1).

Depending on the amount of information applicable to your practice site, basic training will likely take 1 to 2 hours. Advanced training will likely take an additional 1 to 2 hours, which should include a hands-on practice drill for emergency response to adverse vaccine reactions. When your technicians have completed training at each level, provide them with a letter or certificate of achievement to note their success. Recognition of such accomplishments helps build morale.

If technicians' job responsibilities will require them to handle sharps disposal containers and other products that could result in exposure to bloodborne pathogens or other potentially infectious material, annual OSHA training is required. Chapter 17, Infection Control in the Pharmacy Setting, provides more information on the OSHA guidelines.

Roles for Student Pharmacists

If you have the opportunity to collaborate with pharmacy schools, engaging student pharmacists in the immunization delivery service can be a rewarding experience. Students can serve as an information resource when you are implementing or expanding your immunization service.[3] They can perform all of the functions outlined for technicians and, depending on your state's practice act, they may be able to assist with clinical components such as vaccine administration and vaccine counseling. Many states permit students to administer vaccines if they have received training and are directly supervised by pharmacists authorized to administer vaccines. Student pharmacists can also help develop marketing, promotional, and educational materials. Students can be an invaluable resource in the planning and delivery of mass immunization clinics, which are discussed in Chapters 12 and 13.[5,6] Pharmacy practice residents can also be an asset to these clinics.[6] In hospitals and health systems that use standing-order vaccination programs, both students and technicians can be responsible for screening newly admitted patients for vaccine eligibility, assisting pharmacists with documentation, updating patient charts, and educating other health care providers about vaccines.[7] Engaging students in these roles may help to overcome some of the barriers noted by pharmacists (i.e., insufficient time and staff support).[8]

Student pharmacists will appreciate the opportunity to be involved in patient care and to learn a new skill set. With the introductory and advanced pharmacy practice experiences required in all accredited pharmacy curricula, many schools seek additional sites and innovative activities for student pharmacists. Immunization programs and services provide an excellent means to meet the accreditation standards.[9] As a preceptor for these pharmacy practice experiences, you will benefit from the students' assistance in the immunization service and from the chance to teach and positively influence future pharmacists.

References

1. American Society of Health-System Pharmacists. Model Curriculum for Pharmacy Technician Education and Training Programs. 3rd ed. 2013. www.ashp.org/doclibrary/accreditation/model-curriculum.pdf. Accessed October 11, 2014.
2. Ernst ME, Chalstrom CV, Currie JD, et al. Implementation of a community pharmacy-based influenza vaccination program. *J Am Pharm Assoc.* 1997;NS37:570–80.

3. Grabenstein JD. Vaccination roles for pharmacy students. *J Am Pharm Assoc.* 2001;41:344.
4. White paper on pharmacy technicians (2002): needed changes can no longer wait. *J Am Pharm Assoc.* 2003;43:93–104.
5. Dang CJ, Dudley JE, Truong H, et al. Planning and implementation of a student-led immunization clinic. *Am J Pharm Educ.* 2012;7(5):article 78.
6. Conway SE, Johnson EJ, Hagemann TM. Introductory and advanced pharmacy practice experiences within campus-based influenza clinics. *Am J Pharm Educ.* 2013;77(3): article 61.
7. Skledar SJ, McKaveney TP, Sokos DR, et al. Role of student pharmacist interns in a hospital-based standing orders pneumococcal vaccination program. *J Am Pharm Assoc.* 2007;47:404–9.
8. Pace AC, Flowers SK, Hastings JK. Arkansas community pharmacists' opinions on providing immunizations. *J Pharm Pract.* 2010;23:496–501.
9. Soltis D, Flowers SK. Expanding experiential opportunities through patient care services: a focus on immunizations. *J Pharm Pract.* 2010;23:575–8.

Table 11.1

Components of Immunization Service Technician Training

Basic Training

- Rationale for immunizing against vaccine-preventable diseases
  - Overview of the diseases
  - Extent of morbidity and mortality caused by the diseases
- Explanation of the immunization service
  - Timeline for implementation
  - Vaccines to be provided
  - Pricing structures
- Expected outcomes of the service
  - Financial gains
  - Improved customer service
  - Decreased morbidity and mortality
  - Market niche
  - Meeting unmet immunization needs of the community

continued on page 85

- Activities governed by state laws and regulations[1]
  - Tasks to be delegated to technicians
- Roles and responsibilities of pharmacy staff
  - Pharmacists
  - Technicians
  - Student pharmacists, as applicable
  - Ancillary personnel, as applicable
- Billing procedures
  - Out-of-pocket fees
  - Medicare Parts B and D
  - Other third-party insurance providers or employers
- Impact on workflow and operations
  - Processing the vaccine as a prescription
  - Staying organized and efficient
  - Importance of teamwork and communication
- Impact on staff hours
  - Changes to shifts and staffing allocation
- Inventory changes
  - Ordering vaccines
  - Shipping precautions
  - Storage requirements
- Additional precautions that need to be taken by staff
  - Handling syringes and contaminated supplies
  - Process for disposing of sharps and bloodborne pathogens
  - Locating and using the exposure control plan

Advanced Training

All of the components of basic training, plus the following:

- Documentation and patient information
  - Vaccine information statements
  - Screening questionnaires
  - Consent forms, if applicable
  - Documentation of vaccine provided
  - Pharmacy immunization records

continued on page 86

Table 11.1

continued from page 85

- Patient immunization records
- Communicating with other health care providers regarding immunization records

- Scheduling patients and/or clinics
  - Appointment books, electronic calendars, online scheduling
  - Reminder calls
  - Time slots for clinic days
  - Ensuring adequate staff for clinic days
- Marketing the service
  - To patients
  - To health care providers
  - To the community
- Preparing the vaccine supplies
  - Supply list
  - Ensuring the correct patient, correct drug, and correct dose
- Emergency management of vaccine reactions
  - Signs and symptoms of adverse vaccine reactions
  - Emergency supply kit
  - Performing cardiopulmonary resuscitation (CPR)
  - Contacting the emergency medical system (EMS)

Immunization Service and Delivery Options

Chapter 12

Delivery and Workflow Models for Immunization Services

Immunization services may be provided to patients by appointment, on a walk-in basis, or in mass immunization clinics. Each of these delivery models has advantages and disadvantages (Table 12.1).[1–3] Depending on the capabilities of your practice site and the needs of your community, you may be involved in just one delivery model or all three. It will be up to you and your staff to determine which models you will pursue and promote.

If either the appointment or the walk-in model is chosen, the vaccination preparation and delivery process should be aligned with your pharmacy's workflow and dispensing functions. This will minimize disruptions and shorten the patient's wait time. The first step is to ensure that your prescription-processing workflow is organized and free of bottlenecks. The pharmacists should devote their time strictly to patient care and clinical activities while technicians handle all technical dispensing functions. Work stations should be identified and used.[4,5] With these conditions in place, processing vaccine orders should be simple and should coincide efficiently with the prescription-processing workflow. Patient contact time for administering the vaccine can be kept to 5 minutes or less.[6] This is important to keep in mind when factoring in the time it may take to schedule an appointment with a patient. Dr. Jean-Venable "Kelly" R. Goode, Professor at Virginia Commonwealth University School of Pharmacy, has noted that in the time it takes to schedule an appointment with a patient, a vaccine could likely be administered. Coordinating schedules with a patient and placing a reminder call could require more time than would be needed to administer the vaccine on a walk-in basis. If the patient fails to show up for the appointment, then this approach would lead to additional time wasted. Figures 12.1 and 12.2 detail the stepwise processes for vaccinating patients by appointment and on a walk-in basis, respectively.

As noted in Table 12.1, implementing mass immunization clinics requires significant preparation and planning. According to Dr. Stefanie Ferreri,

Clinical Associate Professor at the University of North Carolina Eshelman School of Pharmacy, it typically takes approximately 7 months of planning, with vaccines being ordered in January or February and clinic dates being set in June or July for programs beginning in September. Chapter 13 provides additional guidance on mass immunization clinics that occur off-site. Regardless of location, the following activities must take place during the mass immunization clinic planning process:[3,7]

- Establishing a standing order protocol if one does not exist
- Ordering vaccines and supplies
- Determining the date and time of the event
- Selecting and reserving the location
- Scheduling pharmacists and support staff
- Educating those who will be staffing the event regarding policies, procedures, and responsibilities
- Arranging the physical layout, stations, and flow of traffic to accommodate mass immunization delivery
- Establishing security and emergency procedures
- Setting up a system for record keeping and documentation
- Defining the payment and third-party billing methods to be used
- Communicating with patients, the community, and the media about the event
- Implementing a queue tracking process (e.g., sign-up sheets, numbered cards or tickets) to define and minimize wait times

Dr. Ferreri reports that in her busier clinics, more than 300 patients have been immunized in a 4-hour time period. On slower clinic days, 100 to 150 patients receive immunizations. Typically, over the course of 1 hour, one pharmacist provides immunizations for every 75 to 100 patients. To accommodate this pharmacist-to-patient ratio, two or three pharmacists and three or four technicians or student pharmacists have been assigned to staff the clinic for the 4-hour time period. Pharmacist–patient contact time has been brief, only about 1 minute with each patient.

If it is geographically feasible, Dr. Ferreri recommends partnering with local pharmacy schools to enlist the help of student pharmacists, faculty, and practice residents to meet the staffing needs of mass clinics. The advantages of student pharmacist involvement in mass clinics have also been recognized in an article by Weitzel and Goode.[8] Students from

Virginia Commonwealth University assisted pharmacists and technicians by answering patients' questions. Those in their final year of school administered vaccines under the direct supervision of the pharmacist. As in the other delivery models, the role of the pharmacist in the mass clinic setting should be limited to clinical patient care activities, such as reviewing the screening questions and administering the vaccines.[8] The technicians and student pharmacists, if applicable, should be responsible for processing the initial paperwork, coordinating the flow of traffic, and billing when feasible. They can also assist with the preparatory steps outlined for immunization clinics.

Your first mass immunization clinic will likely present challenges for you and your staff. However, it has the potential to serve as a valuable learning experience. Using a continuous quality improvement (CQI) process, in which you evaluate the successes and pitfalls and make any necessary changes, your next clinic will be more efficient, better organized, and easier to manage. Collecting feedback from your patients and staff will help to guide this CQI process.

References

1. Fontanesi J, Hill L, Olson R, et al. Mass vaccination clinics versus appointments. *J Med Pract Manage.* 2006;21:288–94.
2. Centers for Disease Control and Prevention. Adult immunization programs in nontraditional settings: quality standards and guidance for program evaluation. *MMWR Recomm Rep.* 2000;49(RR-1):1–13.
3. Schwatz B, Worley P. Mass vaccination for annual and pandemic influenza. *Curr Top Microbiol Immunol.* 2006;304:131–52.
4. Angelo LB, Ferreri SP. Assessment of workflow redesign in community pharmacy. *J Am Pharm Assoc.* 2005;45:145–50.
5. Pai AK. Integration of a clinical community pharmacist position: emphasis on workflow redesign. *J Am Pharm Assoc.* 2005;45:400–3.
6. Ernst ME, Chalstrom CV, Currie JD, et al. Implementation of a community pharmacy-based influenza vaccination program. *J Am Pharm Assoc.* 1997;NS37:570–80.
7. Lam AY, Chung Y. Establishing an on-site influenza vaccination service in an assisted-living facility. *J Am Pharm Assoc.* 2008;48:758–63.
8. Weitzel KW, Goode JR. Implementation of a pharmacy-based immunization program in a supermarket chain. *J Am Pharm Assoc.* 2000;40:252–6.

Table 12.1

Comparison of Vaccine Delivery Models

Advantages	Disadvantages
By Appointment	
• Staff can be scheduled according to need • Patient can be screened in advance • Paperwork and prescription can be processed ahead of time • Follow-up appointments are easy to schedule • Patient waiting time is reduced • Type of vaccine available for administration is not limited by on-hand inventory • Beneficial when individual prescription is required for vaccine administration • Allows for adequate patient–provider contact time	• The number of patients who can be vaccinated is limited • Additional staffing resources are needed to maintain appointment book and make reminder calls • Coordinating schedules with patients may present challenges • Appointments may be missed
On a Walk-In Basis	
• Convenient for patients • Increases ability to vaccinate patients who may be at the pharmacy for other reasons (e.g., picking up a prescription, purchasing nonprescription products) • Follow-up appointments are easy to schedule • Allows for adequate patient–provider contact time	• Staffing may not be adequate to accommodate the patient • Vaccine requested may not be in stock • Patient may not be a candidate for the vaccine requested

continued on page 93

In Mass Immunization Clinics

• Simultaneously meets the needs of many patients • Promotes the practice site and service to many individuals • Process is confined to a defined interval of time • Dedicated staff can be allocated for event[1] • Minimal interference with routine pharmacy activities and workflow[1] • Well-suited for seasonal influenza vaccination[2] • Convenient patient access to readily accessible settings[3]	• Preparation process is time-consuming • Additional staff, resources, and space are required • Extensive marketing efforts are needed • May result in long wait times for patients • Limits the types of vaccines available for administration • Patient vaccine records and histories may not be accessible[1] • Relies on patient recall for immunization status[1] • Limits patient–provider contact time • Not feasible if immunization per standing order is not allowed • Storage and temperature monitoring of vaccines can be challenging

Figure 12.1

Vaccine Delivery Workflow for a Patient with an Appointment

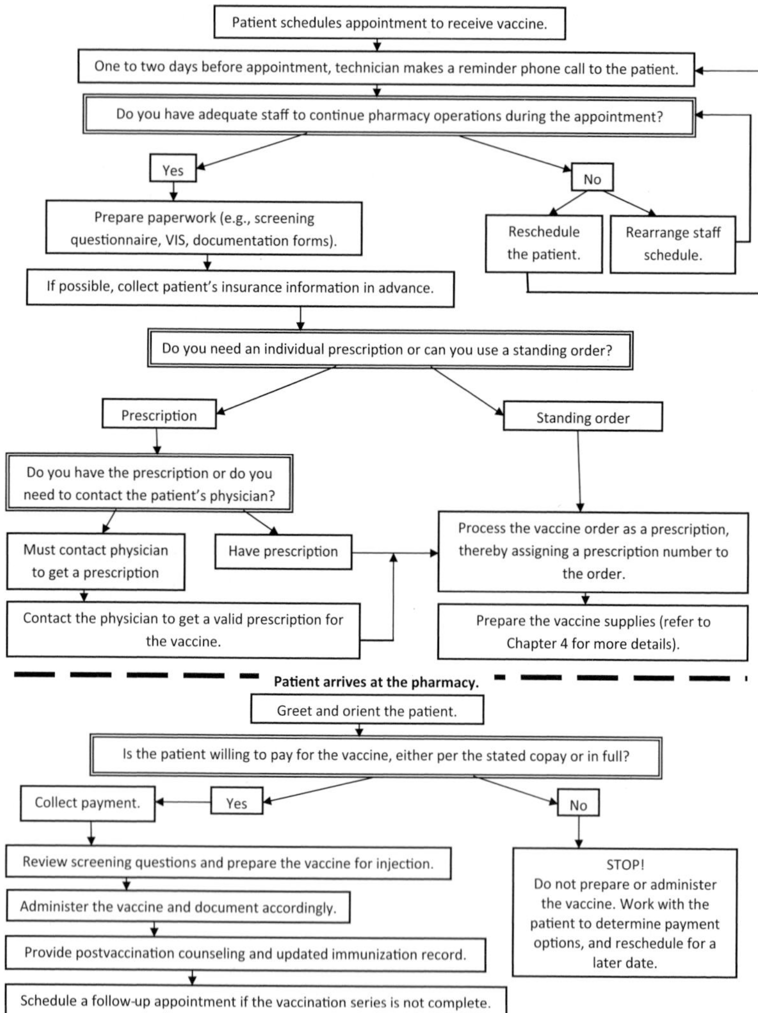

VIS = vaccine information statement.

Figure 12.2

Vaccine Delivery Workflow for a Walk-in Patient

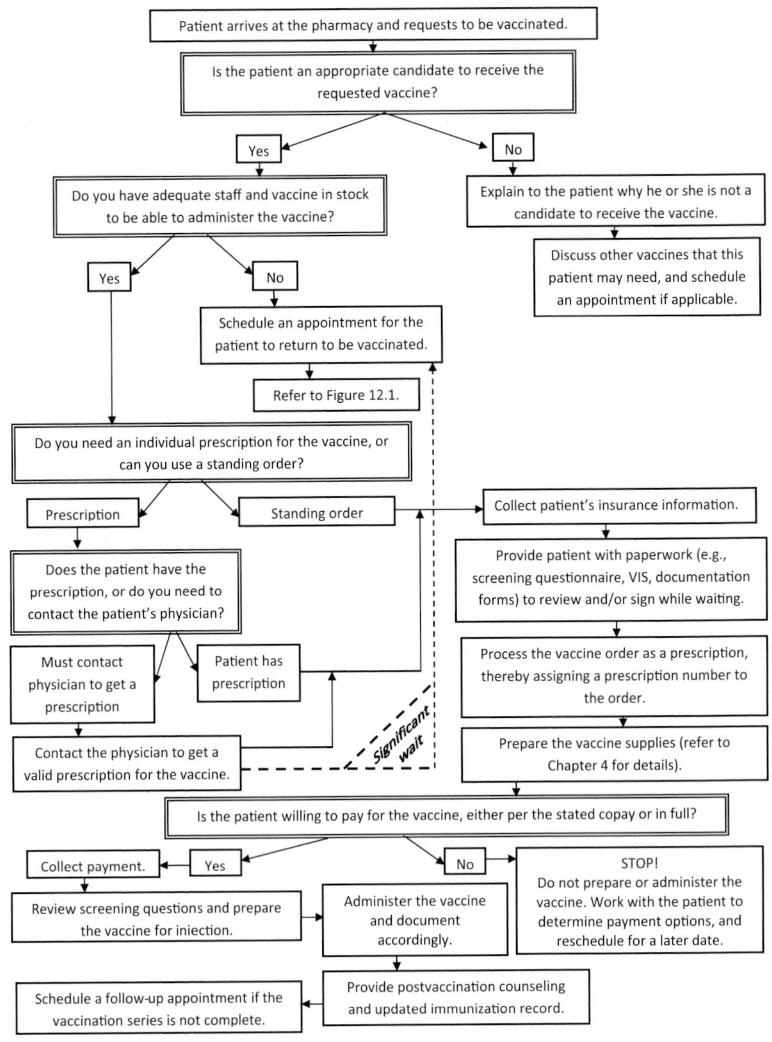

VIS = vaccine information statement.

Chapter 13

Vaccine Delivery in Off-Site Clinics

Immunization providers are often presented with opportunities to vaccinate patients in locations other than their practice sites (e.g., health fairs, community and senior centers, churches, other pharmacies, assisted-living facilities, schools, grocery stores, shopping malls). Providing the service at these venues meets the needs of many patients in the community and can do wonders to improve immunization rates. But planning for such an event is not a simple process. It takes time and dedication. As described in Chapter 12, selecting the site and date and ordering supplies should begin several months in advance. Marketing the event should begin several weeks in advance.

Off-site clinic preparation checklist

- ☐ Order vaccines and supplies
- ☐ Verify that your standing order or protocol will cover off-site immunizations
- ☐ Confirm that your liability insurance covers off-site immunizations (an individual policy is advisable)
- ☐ Visit the site prior to the clinic date to view the facility and meet the site coordinator
- ☐ Determine the location of the nearest restrooms (patients and clinic staff will want to know)
- ☐ Arrange to have the following items set up in advance:
  - o Tables for vaccine providers and patients
  - o Chairs for vaccine providers and patients
  - o Chairs for those waiting to be vaccinated
  - o Waste containers at each vaccination table
- ☐ Design the layout of tables and chairs to allow for efficient traffic flow through the clinic
- ☐ Communicate the desired layout to the facility coordinator
- ☐ Schedule personnel to staff the clinic

continued on page 98

Off-site clinic preparation checklist, *continued from page 97*

- ☐ Assign specific tasks to the clinic staff
- ☐ Post marketing flyers at and near the site
- ☐ Review with the clinic staff immunization, documentation, and emergency management procedures
- ☐ Determine how payment and billing will be managed

The supply list is fairly extensive for off-site immunization clinics. Many of the items that would be readily available at your pharmacy or practice site must be made portable. Plan to purchase several plastic totes or bins to transport the array of supplies.

Supply checklist for off-site clinics

- ☐ Insulated containers or coolers to transport and store vaccine
- ☐ Cold packs
- ☐ Thermometers
- ☐ Temperature log (check hourly)
- ☐ Vaccine for injection
- ☐ Vaccine diluent, as needed to reconstitute lyophilized powders
- ☐ Absorbent pads
- ☐ Adhesive bandages
- ☐ Cotton balls or gauze pads
- ☐ Alcohol swabs
- ☐ Disposable synthetic gloves
- ☐ Hand sanitizer
- ☐ Needles and syringes of varying sizes
- ☐ Sharps disposal containers
- ☐ Biohazard disposal bag
- ☐ Exposure control plan
- ☐ Emergency kit (e.g., epinephrine, epinephrine dosing chart, blood pressure cuffs, stethoscope, CPR barriers or face shields)
- ☐ Cellular phone (to activate emergency medical services)
- ☐ Copy of provider's license
- ☐ Clinical vaccine information resource (for provider use)

continued on page 99

Supply checklist for off-site clinics, *continued from page 98*

- ☐ Clipboards
- ☐ Pens
- ☐ Folders
- ☐ Disposable tablecloths
- ☐ Numbered cards to give to patients (to track the queue)
- ☐ Vaccine information statements
- ☐ Patient intake forms
- ☐ Consent forms, if required
- ☐ Receipts for service that patients can submit for insurance claims
- ☐ Billing roster form if Medicare is to be billed (collect patient information and signature)
- ☐ Immunization record cards to give to patients
- ☐ Educational materials for patients to read or surveys to complete while waiting

In transporting vaccines to your off-site clinic, the cold chain must be maintained at all times.

Recommendations for refrigerated vaccine transport to off-site clinics[1,2]

- Do not place vaccines in the enclosed trunk of a vehicle.
- Use insulated containers capable of maintaining the required vaccine storage temperature. The original vaccine shipping containers, hard-sided insulated plastic coolers, and Styrofoam coolers with 2-inch-thick walls are acceptable. Do not use the thin-walled Styrofoam coolers sold at grocery stores.
- Use conditioned cold packs for refrigerated vaccines. Do not use loose, bagged, or dry ice. A conditioned cold pack is one that has been left at room temperature for 1 to 2 hours until the edges have defrosted and condensation is noticeable.
- Use an insulated barrier (e.g., bubble wrap) between the cold packs and vaccine to avoid freezing.
- Layer the contents of the insulated container starting with the cold packs, then barrier, vaccine, thermometer, another barrier, and additional cold packs.
- Keep vaccines in their original packaging.

continued on page 100

Recommendations for refrigerated vaccine, *continued from page 99*

- Transport diluent for refrigerated vaccines at room temperature, *or* transport it in the same container as the vaccine. If placing the diluent with vaccines, refrigerate it in advance so that the temperature in the container is maintained.
- Label the containers with a "fragile" notation, vaccine description, quantity, date, time, and originating facility.
- During the off-site clinic, monitor and record the temperatures inside the insulated containers hourly with a calibrated thermometer, preferably one with continuous monitoring and recording features. Avoid frequent opening of the containers.
- Ensure that the combined transport and clinic time does not exceed 8 hours.

Transporting vaccines that contain varicella, such as the herpes zoster, varicella, and MMRV (measles, mumps, rubella, and varicella) vaccines, to off-site clinics is not recommended.[2] If such vaccines must be transported for clinic use, they can be stored at refrigerator temperatures (2°C–8°C) for up to 72 hours before reconstitution. Once reconstituted, the vaccines must be used within 30 minutes. Vaccines not used within these intervals must be discarded.

When you are preparing for your off-site clinic and for vaccine transport, emulate the policies and procedures of your state health department. As noted in Chapter 5, prefilling (or predrawing) syringes is not recommended. Vaccine doses should be drawn as they are needed. The alternative is to use prefilled syringes supplied by the manufacturer.[2] However, if providers do predraw syringes, this should be done only during the clinic, and no more than 10 doses or one multidose vial should be predrawn at one time. The individual who predraws the dose should be the same individual who administers the vaccine. When doses are being predrawn, it is important to monitor clinic flow to ensure that all predrawn doses are used. Multidose vials that have been partially used cannot be transferred to another provider or be transported across state lines.[2] Partially used multidose vials can be transported to and from clinics so long as the cold chain is maintained and they are used by the same provider.

Upon returning to your practice site, verify that any unused vaccine has been maintained at the proper temperature at all times before returning it to the refrigerator. Allow ample time to transfer the immunization records from the off-site clinic to your site's documentation system. Submit Medicare billing rosters and forms, as well as any other insurance claims, as applicable.

References

1. California Department of Public Health, Immunization Branch. Transporting refrigerated vaccine. September 2014. www.eziz.org/assets/docs/IMM-983.pdf. Accessed October 11, 2014.
2. Centers for Disease Control and Prevention. Vaccine Storage and Handling Toolkit. May 2014. www.cdc.gov/vaccines/recs/storage/toolkit/storage-handling-toolkit.pdf. Accessed October 11, 2014.

Chapter 14

Travel Health and Vaccination Clinics

Some pharmacists who provide routine immunizations may wish to take their services a step further by venturing into travel health. Providing travel recommendations and vaccines can be a very rewarding experience—professionally and financially. Patient satisfaction with pharmacy-based travel health services has been high.[1,2] This chapter provides a brief overview of the steps necessary to be a travel health expert. If this is an area of interest for you, you will need to consult additional resources (see Table 14.1) before implementing a travel health and vaccination service.

Offering a travel health service entails much more than the administration of vaccines. You must serve as an information resource for patients, travel companies, and other health care providers. You will need to be able to evaluate your patient's risks according to the details of his or her travel plans. Factors to evaluate include the patient's medication history, diseases endemic in the area, patient's intended activities and quality of lodging, season of the year, altitude, mode of travel, and vaccine needs.[3,4] The traveler's itinerary and changes in the itinerary are also important, as vaccination requirements may differ depending on the most recent country visited. Two books you will find particularly useful as you begin to educate yourself about travel health and vaccines are

- *CDC Health Information for International Travel 2014* (Yellow Book) by the Centers for Disease Control and Prevention, and
- *International Travel and Health 2012* by the World Health Organization.

Both of these publications are available online free of charge and are updated routinely.

A wide array of print materials for patients and providers is available from multiple organizations (Table 14.1). It is important to be familiar with these websites and the type of education offered. It may be beneficial to obtain the Certificate in Travel Health from the International Society of Travel Medicine. You will need to be able to recognize your own limitations and refer patients to a travel medicine expert when appropriate.[3]

Included in your travel health service should be recommendations for the prevention and management of ailments, conditions, and health risks common to international travel, such as the following:[3,5,6]

- Altitude and motion sickness
- Animal-associated hazards
- Bacterial skin infections
- Chikungunya
- Cholera
- Deep-vein thrombosis and pulmonary embolism
- Dehydration
- Dengue fever
- Diarrhea
- Food and water safety
- Giardiasis
- Jet lag
- Insect avoidance and protection
- Leishmaniasis
- Malaria
- Management of chronic disease during travel
- Schistosomiasis
- Sexually transmitted diseases
- Sunburn (this should include a review of the patient's medications for any with photosensitivity precautions)
- Temperature extremes
- Vaccine-preventable diseases

Depending on the patient's travel destination, you may need to recommend certain nonprescription and prescription products to prevent or treat such conditions. All patients should travel with a medical kit consisting of first-aid supplies and any recommended prescription and nonprescription medications.[5]

Patients with chronic disease (e.g., hypertension, diabetes, asthma, chronic obstructive pulmonary disease, HIV infection, coronary artery disease, rheumatoid arthritis, epilepsy) should be instructed on managing their conditions during travel, as follows:

- They should have enough medication to last the duration of the trip plus a few extra days to account for travel-related delays.
- They may need to request a vacation override from their insurance provider to acquire enough medication to last the duration of the trip.
- They should work with you and their physicians to ensure that their conditions are stable before travel begins.
- They may want to purchase travel health insurance.
- They should know in advance whom to contact and where to go in the event of an emergency.
- They should obtain a letter from their physicians certifying the need for their respective medications.

Travel health recommendations for patients with special needs (i.e., infants, children, pregnant or breast-feeding women, and immuno-compromised patients) are beyond the scope of this chapter. Consult the resources noted in this chapter for more information on these specific groups of travelers.

Vaccines recommended or required for travel vary by destination. They may include vaccines against Japanese encephalitis, rabies (pre-exposure), typhoid, and yellow fever (Table 14.2), along with other vaccines routinely recommended by ACIP.[3,7–12] According to the International Health Regulations, only approved sites can distribute and administer yellow fever vaccine.[12] State health departments are responsible for certifying providers and sites. This information is reported to CDC for inclusion in the U.S. Yellow Fever Vaccination Center Registry.

Refer to your state practice act to determine what vaccines you are allowed to administer. If permitted, you may wish to expand your service to include the administration of travel vaccines. The stepwise process for working with a patient planning to travel internationally is detailed as follows.

Planning to meet with your patient:

- Schedule an appointment with your patient 4 to 6 weeks before travel is to begin.

- Determine your patient's planned destination, length of stay, season of travel, accommodations, and intended activities.
- Research the recommendations and risks for the destination.
- Determine what vaccines and other health precautions your patient will need.
- Print any applicable patient education information to review during the appointment.
- Prepare global maps to review with your patient.

During the appointment:

- Review the patient's medication and vaccination history.
- Outline any routine and travel vaccinations that are either required or recommended for your patient's destination.
- Describe the signs and symptoms of diseases endemic to the area.
- Discuss prescription and nonprescription medications, as well as supplies, that your patient will need.
- Explain the importance and proper use of infection control measures, including hand and cough hygiene.
- Assist your patient in preparing a travel medication kit.
- Provide your patient with a travel checklist, with items specific to your patient's travel clearly marked.

If you are able to administer travel vaccines:

- Contact your patient's physician to get prescriptions for medications and vaccines.
- Schedule the appointment to administer vaccines.
- When applicable, provide your patient with the International Certificate of Vaccination or Prophylaxis, which is required for proof of yellow fever vaccination.
- Discuss any incomplete vaccination series that will need to be addressed upon your patient's return.

Once you are ready to provide your travel health service, you will need to let others know what the service will entail and the value it has for travelers. Work with travel agencies in your area. Let them know about the services you offer and encourage them to refer customers to you for a vaccine needs assessment. Discuss your service with physicians and office staff in your community. Collaborate with other pharmacists who do not specialize in this area for referrals. Provide these individuals and groups with marketing materials as well as referral cards containing your contact information. Refer to Chapter 9 for guidance on marketing your service.

References

1. Hess KM, Dai CW, Garner B, et al. Measuring outcomes of a pharmacist-run travel health clinic located in an independent community pharmacy. *J Am Pharm Assoc.* 2010;50(2):174–80.
2. Gatewood SB, Stanley DD, Goode JV. Implementation of a comprehensive pretravel health program in a supermarket chain pharmacy. *J Am Pharm Assoc.* 2009;49(5):660–9.
3. Centers for Disease Control and Prevention. *CDC Health Information for International Travel 2014.* New York: Oxford University Press; 2013.
4. American Pharmacists Association. Pharmacy-Based Immunization Delivery: A National Certificate Program for Pharmacists. 11th ed. Washington, DC: American Pharmacists Association; 2009.
5. American Pharmacists Association. The One Minute Counselor: A pharmacist's guide to travel health and vaccinations. 2007. www.pharmacist.com/AM/Template.cfm?Section=One_Minute_Counselors&. Accessed July 16, 2011.
6. Goad JA, Stanley DD. Strategies for implementing a pharmacy-based travel health and vaccine service—2008 update: a multimedia CE program for pharmacists. American Pharmacists Association Continuing Education.
7. *International Travel and Health 2012.* Geneva, Switzerland: World Health Organization; 2012.
8. IXIARO [package insert]. Livingston, UK: Intercell Biomedical; 2013.
9. Vivotif [package insert]. Berne, Switzerland: Crucell Vaccines, Inc.; 2013.
10. Typhim Vi [package insert]. Lyon, France: Sanofi Pasteur; 2014.
11. YF-VAX [package insert]. Swiftwater, PA: Sanofi Pasteur; 2013.
12. Centers for Disease Control and Prevention. Yellow fever vaccine: recommendations of the Advisory Committee on Immunization Practices (ACIP). *MMWR.* 2010;59(RR-7).

Table 14.1

Travel Health and Vaccination Resources

CDC Traveler's Health • *CDC Health Information for International Travel* (Yellow Book) • Vaccine recommendations • Disease information • Travel clinic locator • Travel notices • Continuing education courses and training • Destination-specific information • Guidance for specific groups • Mobile apps • RSS feeds for automatic updates	wwwnc.cdc.gov/travel
WHO International Travel and Health • *International Travel and Health 2012* • Updates for travelers • Safe food guidance • International Health Regulations • WHO International Certificate of Vaccination or Prophylaxis information	www.who.int/ith/en
International Society of Travel Medicine • Certificate in Travel Health continuing professional development program • Travel clinic locator • News and updates • Travel medicine meetings and conferences	www.istm.org
The American Society of Tropical Medicine and Hygiene • Certificate of Knowledge in Clinical Tropical Medicine and Travelers' Health • Tropical medicine resources and education • Meeting information	www.astmh.org
Immunization Action Coalition International Travel • Patient handouts • Links to other travel resources	www.immunize.org/travel

Table 14.2

Overview of Select Travel-Related Diseases and Vaccines[a]

Disease	Disease and Vaccine Information
Japanese encephalitis	• Transmitted by mosquitoes • Occurs primarily in rural agricultural areas where flooding irrigation is practiced, primarily in Asia • Vaccination is not recommended for travel lasting less than 1 month and is restricted to urban areas or when it is not a JE virus transmission season • JE-VC vaccine (IXIARO, Intercell Biomedical) is an inactivated vaccine administered intramuscularly as a two-dose series given 28 days apart for travelers older than 2 months of age • The series should be completed at least 1 week before travel to allow for adequate immune response and monitoring of adverse effects • A booster dose may be administered after at least 1 year for travelers age 17 and older, if needed
Rabies	• Transmitted via contact with rabid animals • Present in most countries • Most common transmission in developing countries is via dog bites; transmission is also related to bat bites in any country • Preexposure vaccination is limited to those who are at significant risk of exposure or will be without access to modern rabies vaccine • Two vaccine formulations: human diploid cell vaccine (Imovax, Sanofi Pasteur) and purified chick embryo cell vaccine (RabAvert, Novartis) • Three injections (at 0, 7, and 21 or 28 days) must be complete before travel • Postexposure prophylaxis is recommended even if a preexposure vaccine was given, but the administration protocol is different

continued on page 110

Table 14.2

continued from page 109

Typhoid fever	• Transmitted primarily via the fecal–oral route (e.g., food or water contaminated with infected fecal matter) • Common in areas with poor sanitation and food preparation measures • Exists worldwide • Highest risk exists in South Asia; other areas of risk include East and Southeast Asia, Africa, the Caribbean, and Central and South America • Two formulations exist: live attenuated typhoid Ty21a vaccine given orally (Vivotif, Berna) and inactivated typhoid Vi polysaccharide vaccine given intramuscularly (Typhim Vi, Sanofi Pasteur) • Live vaccine is for travelers age 6 and older; one capsule is given every 48 hours for a total of four doses, with a four-dose booster every 5 years if needed • Inactivated vaccine is for travelers age 2 and older; 1 dose is given with a booster every 2 years if needed

continued on page 111

Yellow fever	• Transmitted by mosquitoes • Exists in sub-Saharan Africa and tropical South America • Vaccine (YF-VAX, Sanofi Pasteur) is a live attenuated virus given subcutaneously to travelers 9 months and older, with a booster every 10 years if needed • Contraindicated in travelers less than 6 months of age, and carries a precaution due to increased risk of adverse effects for those age 6–8 months and those 60 years and older • Pregnant and breast-feeding women should avoid the vaccine if possible • Yellow fever vaccine is required to enter certain countries; the Certificate of Vaccination is not valid until 10 days after vaccination • Distribution of vaccine is limited to approved sites

[a]Routine vaccines (e.g., hepatitis A, Hib, influenza, measles, meningococcal, polio, Td/Tdap, varicella) or booster doses may be recommended or required depending on destination.
Source: References 3, 7–12.

Safety Measures

Chapter 15

Prevention and Management of Adverse Events and Emergencies

Vaccines, like medications or medical products, can result in adverse reactions. Serious adverse events or complications from vaccines are extremely rare. Still, each patient should be evaluated for potential precautions or contraindications in order to reduce the risk of adverse effects, events, and complications from vaccines.[1]

Precautions are conditions that may hinder the patient's response to a vaccine or increase the patient's risk of an adverse reaction.[2] *Contraindications* are conditions that will likely result in a severe, life-threatening event if the patient receives the vaccine.[2] When a contraindication exists, the risks outweigh the benefits and the vaccine should not be given.[2] If a precaution exists, it is your responsibility to ensure that the risks and benefits to the patient are fully evaluated before the vaccine is administered. When a precaution is identified, contact the patient's primary care provider to collaboratively determine the next course of action for the patient. In most cases, the vaccine can be given at a later time.[2]

As an immunization provider, you can take the following steps to help ensure that the vaccines you administer to your patients are safe and effective:[3]

- Store and administer vaccines as recommended by the manufacturer and CDC.
- Adhere to the timing and spacing requirements for vaccine doses.
- Observe the precautions and contraindications noted for each vaccine.
- Properly manage adverse vaccine effects and events.
- Report suspected adverse vaccine reactions to the Vaccine Adverse Event Reporting System (VAERS).
- Educate patients and caregivers regarding the benefits and risks of vaccines.

Screening Questions

To help you evaluate whether or not precautions or contraindications exist for each patient, a series of screening questions should be asked. If a patient responds affirmatively to any of the questions, it does not necessarily mean that the vaccine cannot be given. Rather, additional information needs to be obtained to determine if and when the vaccine can be administered. The Immunization Action Coalition (IAC) suggests specific screening questions and recommended actions when patients respond affirmatively.[4,5] This information can be found at www.immunize.org/handouts/screening-vaccines.asp and is summarized in Table 15.1. The contraindications and precautions for each vaccine can be found in Chapter 19.

Vaccine Information Statements

Patients should be given reliable and accurate information about the inherent risks and benefits associated with vaccines prior to administration. The National Childhood Vaccine Injury Act (NCVIA) passed in 1986 changed the vaccine safety responsibilities of health care providers in several ways.[6] All health care providers who administer certain vaccines must provide patients or caregivers with vaccine information statements (VISs). Developed by CDC for patients and caregivers, VISs contain information regarding the benefits and adverse events associated with each vaccine.[7,8] Under federal law (NCVIA), the patient or caregiver must be given the current VIS before receiving any of the vaccines or components listed in the Vaccine Injury Table (Table 15.2), which include the following:

- Diphtheria
- Haemophilus influenzae type B (Hib)
- Hepatitis A
- Hepatitis B
- Influenza
- Human papillomavirus
- Measles
- Meningococcal
- Mumps
- Pertussis
- Pneumococcal conjugate
- Polio

- Rotavirus
- Rubella
- Tetanus
- Varicella

The date the VIS was provided, as well as the publication date of the VIS, must be noted in the patient's chart or medical record. If you are administering a combination vaccine for which a VIS is not available, you must provide a VIS for each component of the vaccine.

VISs are also available for the other vaccines not listed here. Although you are not legally required to distribute them, it is highly recommended that you do. VISs can be obtained from the IAC or CDC websites. VISs are available in more than 30 languages from IAC.

Patients with mobile devices have the option of downloading VISs as opposed to receiving paper copies. Refer patients who choose this option to www.cdc.gov/vaccines/hcp/vis/mobile.html and ensure that they click the link for the appropriate VIS. You will still need to record the VIS publication date and the date the VIS was downloaded.

Vaccine Adverse Event and Error Reporting Systems

Health care providers are required to report to VAERS certain adverse events resulting from vaccination.[6] The NCVIA requires reporting of any event that is either listed by the vaccine manufacturer as a contraindication to subsequent doses or included in the Vaccine Injury Table and occurring within the specified time period.[9] The Vaccine Injury Table (Table 15.2) lists events that may be associated with a vaccine and the time interval in which the event would need to occur to be vaccine related.[10] If a patient experiences an adverse event not listed in this table, you are still encouraged to report it. All clinically significant adverse events should be reported, even if causality cannot be determined.[9]

Reporting to VAERS enables postmarketing data and surveillance on adverse events after vaccine administration to be captured and analyzed. The VAERS form collects the following information: (1) person reporting the event, (2) patient, (3) vaccine administration, (4) adverse event and event outcomes, and (5) vaccines, medication, and prior adverse events. Reporting can be done either electronically or on paper; forms for reporting can be found at http://vaers.hhs.gov/esub/index.

If an error occurs either before or during vaccine administration, this should be reported to the Vaccine Error Reporting Program, located at http://verp.ismp.org. Examples of such errors include wrong vaccine, wrong time or interval, wrong route, wrong patient, wrong dose, wrong age, wrong site, expired vaccine, contaminated vaccine, diluent given without the vaccine, and missing component of a multicomponent vaccine. The reporting and tracking of vaccine administration errors serves as an important mechanism for educating others and preventing such errors from recurring.

Management of Adverse Events

Your cardiopulmonary resuscitation (CPR) certification should be current before you begin to administer vaccines. All pharmacy staff involved in vaccine delivery need to take a course intended for health care providers. Numerous organizations offer CPR training; the American Heart Association and the American Red Cross are two reputable organizations that offer CPR training for health care providers. Both provide search engines for locating classes and facilities in your area. For classes affiliated with the American Heart Association, go to www.americanheart.org and click on "CPE & ECC." For classes affiliated with the American Red Cross, go to www.redcross.org and click on "Training & Certification."

You have the option to offer CPR courses at your workplace. You or another staff person, such as one of your more experienced technicians, could become a certified instructor and teach the courses to other pharmacy personnel. Larger companies or organizations employing numerous individuals for whom routine CPR certification is required might find this to be a wise investment.

As noted in Chapters 5 and 6, you should have protocols established for medical management of adverse reactions to vaccines and have an emergency supply kit available. It is critical that you and your staff be familiar with the protocols and proper use of the emergency supplies

(Table 15.3). The stepwise process that you and your staff will implement in the event of a vaccine-related emergency should be recorded in writing and should be rehearsed. Telephone access for contacting emergency medical services (EMS) should be available at all locations where vaccines are provided.

The approach to patient care and management will vary depending on the type of adverse reaction (Table 15.4).[11] Vasovagal syncope, or fainting, is more common than anaphylaxis and has a higher prevalence among adolescents and young adults.[2] Avoiding injury due to falls is a primary concern in syncopal episodes. Administering vaccines in a safe environment and observing the patient after vaccination are critical. For anaphylaxis, the use of epinephrine should be first-line treatment. Diphenhydramine, an H1-receptor antagonist, may be used as second-line therapy.[11–13] Some state practice acts and health department protocols may recommend or even require the use of diphenhydramine as part of the emergency treatment plan. When developing your emergency protocol, you will need to determine whether diphenhydramine is required. Some providers may also administer injectable ranitidine, an H2-receptor antagonist, as adjunct second-line therapy with diphenhydramine. However, using ranitidine in this manner is not a common practice for pharmacists in outpatient settings.

The adolescent and adult dose of epinephrine (1:1000) ranges from 0.3 to 0.5 mg, with a maximum single dose of 0.5 mg.[11,12] For infants and children, the epinephrine dose is based on weight (0.01 mg/kg), with a maximum single dose of 0.3 mg.[12,13] It is administered intramuscularly every 5 to 20 minutes, if needed, for up to three doses.[2,12,13] Epinephrine should be administered in the anterolateral aspect of the thigh or at the vaccine injection site in the deltoid muscle, which may help to slow vaccine absorption.[2,12] Do not administer epinephrine in the buttocks, which could lead to delayed or erratic absorption, or near the extremities, which could result in diminished blood flow and necrosis. To reduce the risk of dosing errors with epinephrine, use caution when ordering epinephrine ampuls, and stock only the 1:1000 (1 mg/mL) concentration if possible. If you must stock multiple epinephrine concentrations, apply auxiliary warning labels to the vials to alert staff of the different concentrations.[14] If you are using an epinephrine autoinjector and administering the drug into the anterolateral aspect of the thigh, you will need to exert force to ensure that the needle enters the muscle. With the autoinjector, the injection can be given through clothing.

The standard pediatric dose of diphenhydramine is 1–2 mg/kg every 4 to 6 hours, with a maximum single dose of 30 mg for children and 50 mg for adolescents.[12,13] Adults can be given 1–2 mg/kg or 25–50 mg of diphenhydramine every 4 to 6 hours, with a maximum single dose of 100 mg.[11,12] Diphenhydramine can be given orally or by intramuscular or intravenous injection as second-line therapy for anaphylaxis and may be beneficial if hives or pruritus accompanies the attack.[12] Although administration by injection is preferred, oral diphenhydramine may be effective for milder attacks.[11] Oral solutions may have a faster onset of action than tablets.[15] However, pharmacists will need to carefully consider giving a medication by the oral route to a patient having an anaphylactic reaction; this may cause further complications for patients experiencing facial swelling or breathing difficulties.

Refer to the simplified dosing tables (Tables 15.5 and 15.6)[13,16–20] for suggested weight-based dosing of epinephrine and diphenhydramine. Dosing tables should be included in your emergency supply kit.

Emergency preparedness tips for vaccinating infants and children

- The CPR certification course you select should include infant and child CPR.[21]
- The emergency supply kit should contain needles, syringes, blood pressure cuffs, and CPR barriers or face shields of appropriate sizes for infants and children.
- Dosing of epinephrine and diphenhydramine is based on weight. Document the child's weight *before* administering the vaccine.

If a syncopal or anaphylactic episode is going to occur, it will likely take place within minutes of the vaccination. Therefore, CDC recommends that providers observe patients for at least 15 minutes following the vaccination.[2] It can be challenging to keep patients in the pharmacy or at the vaccination site for 15 minutes. Some activities to keep patients occupied during this time include the following:

- Filling out a satisfaction survey
- Working with pharmacy staff to complete their immunization records
- Scheduling appointments for follow-up vaccinations
- Reading a brochure or educational information about other services offered at the pharmacy
- Signing up for your pharmacy's electronic mailing list or newsletter (If you institute an electronic mailing list, you must blind carbon copy (BCC) the recipients to protect patient privacy.)
- Receiving a complimentary blood pressure or body composition assessment (Avoid taking a blood pressure measurement in the arm used for the vaccination.)

References

1. American Pharmacists Association. Pharmacy-Based Immunization Delivery: A National Certificate Program for Pharmacists. 11th ed. Washington, DC: American Pharmacists Association; 2009.
2. Centers for Disease Control and Prevention. General recommendations on immunization: recommendations of the Advisory Committee on Immunization Practices (ACIP) [published correction appears in *MMWR Recomm Rep.* 2011;60:993]. *MMWR Recomm Rep.* 2011;60(RR-2):1–64.
3. Centers for Disease Control and Prevention. *Epidemiology and Prevention of Vaccine-Preventable Diseases.* Atkinson W, Wolfe S, Hamborsky J, eds. 12th ed (2nd printing, May 2012). Washington, DC: Public Health Foundation; 2011.
4. Immunization Action Coalition. Screening questionnaire for adult immunization. www.immunize.org/catg.d/p4065.pdf. Accessed December 11, 2014.
5. Immunization Action Coalition. Screening questionnaire for child and teen immunization. www.immunize.org/catg.d/p4060.pdf. Accessed December 11, 2014.
6. Centers for Disease Control and Prevention. History of vaccine safety. www.cdc.gov/vaccinesafety/Vaccine_Monitoring/history.html. Accessed October 12, 2014.
7. Immunization Action Coalition. It's federal law! You must give your patients current Vaccine Information Statements (VISs). www.immunize.org/catg.d/p2027.pdf. Accessed October 12, 2014.
8. Vaccine information. 42 CFR § 300aa–26 (1989).
9. Vaccine Adverse Event Reporting System. Information for healthcare professionals. http://vaers.hhs.gov/professionals/index. Accessed October 12, 2014.
10. Health Resources and Services Administration. National Vaccine Injury Compensation Program. Vaccine injury table. www.hrsa.gov/vaccinecompensation/vaccinetable.html. Accessed October 12, 2014.

11. Immunization Action Coalition. Medical management of vaccine reactions in adult patients. www.immunize.org/catg.d/p3082.pdf. Accessed October 12, 2014.
12. Lieberman P, Nicklas RA, Oppenheimer J, et al. The diagnosis and management of anaphylaxis practice parameter: 2010 update. *J Allergy Clin Immunol.* 2010;126: 477–80.e42.
13. Immunization Action Coalition. Medical management of vaccine reactions in children and teens. www.immunize.org/catg.d/p3082a.pdf. Accessed October 12, 2014.
14. Institute for Safe Medication Practices. ISMP advocates changes in epinephrine labeling [press release]. August 12, 2004. www.ismp.org/pressroom/PR20040812.pdf. Accessed October 12, 2014.
15. Boyce JA, Assa'ad A, Burks AW, et al. Guidelines for the diagnosis and management of food allergy in the United States: report of the NIAID-sponsored expert panel. *J Allergy Clin Immunol.* 2010;126:S1–S58.
16. Adrenaclick [package insert]. Atlanta, GA: Sciele Pharma; October 2009.
17. Auvi-Q [package insert]. Bridgewater, NJ: Sanofi-Aventis; February 2014.
18. EpiPen and EpiPen Jr [package insert]. Napa, CA: Dey, LP; September 2008.
19. Twinject [package insert]. Atlanta, GA: Shionogi Pharma; January 2010.
20. Epinephrine injection, USP [package insert]. Peapack, NJ: Greenstone LLC; January 2010.
21. Gardner JS. A practical guide to establishing vaccine administration services in community pharmacies. *J Am Pharm Assoc.* 1997;NS37:683–93.

Table 15.1

Screening Questions and Recommendations[a]

Is the patient sick today?

Even though no evidence exists to indicate that acute illness can reduce efficacy or increase adverse events, it is recommended that vaccines be delayed if a patient has a moderate or severe acute illness. A patient who has a mild illness such as otitis media, a mild upper respiratory infection, or gastrointestinal illness (i.e., diarrhea) or is taking antibiotics can still be vaccinated.

Is the patient allergic to medications, food, a vaccine component, or latex?

An anaphylactic reaction following a previous dose of vaccine or exposure to vaccine components is a contraindication, and the patient should not be vaccinated. A local reaction is not a contraindication. Development of hives or other serious reactions after eating eggs may not necessarily preclude vaccination with inactivated influenza vaccine; consult ACIP recommendations for additional guidance. Consult Appendix B in the CDC's *Epidemiology and Prevention of Vaccine-Preventable Diseases* (the Pink Book) regarding latex and other excipients used in vaccines and vaccine packaging.

Has the patient had a serious reaction to a vaccine?

An anaphylactic reaction following a previous dose of vaccine or exposure to vaccine components is a contraindication, and the patient should not be vaccinated. Consult the Advisory Committee on Immunization Practices (ACIP) recommendations and product package inserts for other adverse events resulting from vaccination that may also constitute contraindications or precautions.

Does the patient have asthma, lung disease, heart disease, kidney disease, a metabolic or endocrine disorder (e.g., diabetes), or a blood disorder?

This question should be used for patients requesting the influenza vaccine. The live attenuated influenza vaccine (LAIV) is contraindicated for persons with these conditions. A patient with these conditions should receive the trivalent inactivated influenza vaccine (TIV).

continued on page 124

Table 15.1

continued from page 123

If the patient is less than 18 years of age, is the patient receiving aspirin therapy?
This question should be used for patients needing the influenza vaccine. The live attenuated influenza vaccine (LAIV) is contraindicated in children and adolescents receiving aspirin therapy because of the risk of Reye's syndrome. These individuals should receive the trivalent inactivated influenza vaccine (TIV).

If the patient is between the ages of 2 and 4 years, has he or she experienced wheezing or been diagnosed with asthma in the past 12 months?
This question should be used for children needing the influenza vaccine. The live attenuated influenza vaccine (LAIV) is contraindicated for persons with these conditions. A child with these conditions should receive the trivalent inactivated influenza vaccine (TIV).

If the child is a candidate for rotavirus vaccine, has the child ever had intussusception?
Infants with a history of intussusception should not be given rotavirus vaccine.

Does the patient have a seizure, brain, or other nervous system disorder?
This question applies to patients requesting DTaP, Td, Tdap, MMRV (measles, mumps, rubella, and varicella), or influenza vaccines. Do not administer DTaP or Tdap to patients who have experienced encephalopathy within 7 days of receiving DTP/DTaP administered before the age of 7 years. If the patient's neurologic disorder is stable and not related to vaccination, the patient can be vaccinated. Children requesting MMRV with a personal or family (i.e., parent or sibling) history of seizures should receive MMR (measles, mumps, and rubella) and VAR (varicella) separately. If a patient requesting Td, Tdap, or influenza vaccine has a history of Guillain-Barré syndrome, consult the ACIP recommendations and the patient's primary care provider. The decision to vaccinate should be based on a risk–benefit analysis.

Does the patient have cancer, leukemia, HIV or AIDS, or any other disease that affects the immune system?
This question applies to live virus vaccines. In general, immunocompromised patients should not receive live virus vaccines. Some exceptions exist. Consult

continued on page 125

current ACIP recommendations and the patient's primary care provider before administering a live vaccine.

Has the patient taken corticosteroids, anticancer medication, or other immunosuppressive therapy or received radiation treatment in the past 3 months?
This question applies to live virus vaccines. These vaccines should be deferred for at least 1 month after discontinuation of high-dose systemic corticosteroid therapy administered for longer than 2 weeks.[2] Consult current ACIP recommendations for specific guidance regarding the length of time to postpone vaccines after chemotherapy or other immunosuppressive therapy.

Has the patient received a blood transfusion or been given blood products, immune globulin, or antiviral medications in the past year?
This question applies to live virus vaccines. Blood products can inhibit the immune response to the measles and rubella vaccines for at least 3 months.[2] Consult current ACIP recommendations for specific intervals. Antiviral influenza medications can reduce the effectiveness of LAIV if given less than 48 hours prior to or within 14 days following LAIV vaccination.[2] Antiviral medications used against herpes may reduce the effectiveness of varicella and zoster vaccines if given less than 24 hours before or within 14 days after these vaccines.[2]

Is the patient pregnant or is there a chance she could become pregnant in the next month?
This question applies to live virus vaccines. There is a theoretical risk of virus transmission to the fetus if a live vaccine is given 1 month prior to or during pregnancy. Avoid the inactivated poliovirus vaccine during pregnancy unless the risk of disease is high. Inactivated influenza virus vaccine (IIV) and Tdap are recommended during pregnancy.

Has the patient received any vaccines in the past 4 weeks?
This question applies to live virus vaccines. Patients who receive a live vaccine should wait at least 28 days before receiving another live vaccine, unless both are administered on the same day. Inactivated vaccines may be given without regard to timing of live vaccine administration.

[a]Screening questionnaires specific for ages and influenza vaccination can be found at www.immunize.org/handouts/screening-vaccines.asp.
Adapted from: References 4 and 5.

Table 15.2

National Childhood Vaccine Injury Act Vaccine Injury Table[a,b]

Vaccine	Illness, Disability, Injury, or Condition Covered	Time Period[c]
I. Vaccines containing tetanus toxoid (e.g., DTaP, DTP, DT, Td, or TT)	A. Anaphylaxis or anaphylactic shock	4 hours
	B. Brachial neuritis	2–28 days
	C. Any acute complication or sequela (including death) of an illness, disability, injury, or condition referred to above, which illness, disability, injury, or condition arose within the time period prescribed	Not applicable
II. Vaccines containing whole cell pertussis bacteria, extracted or partial cell pertussis bacteria, or specific pertussis antigen(s) (e.g., DTP, DTaP, P, DTP-Hib)	A. Anaphylaxis or anaphylactic shock	4 hours
	B. Encephalopathy (or encephalitis)	72 hours
	C. Any acute complication or sequela (including death) of an illness, disability, injury, or condition referred to above, which illness, disability, injury, or condition arose within the time period prescribed	Not applicable
III. Measles, mumps, and rubella vaccine or any of its components (e.g., MMR, MR, M, R)	A. Anaphylaxis or anaphylactic shock	4 hours
	B. Encephalopathy (or encephalitis)	5–15 days (not less than 5 days and not more than 15 days)
	C. Any acute complication or sequela (including death) of an illness, disability, injury, or condition referred to above, which illness, disability, injury, or condition arose within the time period prescribed	Not applicable

continued on page 127

IV. Vaccines containing rubella virus (e.g., MMR, MR, R)	A. Chronic arthritis	7–42 days
	B. Any acute complication or sequela (including death) of an illness, disability, injury, or condition referred to above, which illness, disability, injury, or condition arose within the time period prescribed	Not applicable
V. Vaccines containing measles virus (e.g., MMR, MR, M)	A. Thrombocytopenic purpura	7–30 days
	B. Vaccine-strain measles viral infection in an immunodeficient recipient	6 months
	C. Any acute complication or sequela (including death) of an illness, disability, injury, or condition referred to above, which illness, disability, injury, or condition arose within the time period prescribed	Not applicable
VI. Vaccines containing polio live virus (OPV)	A. Paralytic polio —in a non-immunodeficient recipient	30 days
	—in an immunodeficient recipient	6 months
	—in a vaccine-associated community case	Not applicable
	B. Vaccine-strain polio viral infection —in a non-immunodeficient recipient	30 days
	—in an immunodeficient recipient	6 months
	—in a vaccine-associated community case	Not applicable
	C. Any acute complication or sequela (including death) of an illness, disability, injury, or condition referred to above, which illness, disability, injury, or condition arose within the time period prescribed	Not applicable

continued on page 128

Table 15.2

continued from page 127

Vaccine	Illness, Disability, Injury, or Condition Covered	Time Period[c]
VII. Vaccines containing polio inactivated virus (e.g., IPV)	A. Anaphylaxis or anaphylactic shock	4 hours
	B. Any acute complication or sequela (including death) of an illness, disability, injury, or condition referred to above, which illness, disability, injury, or condition arose within the time period prescribed	Not applicable
VIII. Hepatitis B. vaccines	A. Anaphylaxis or anaphylactic shock	4 hours
	B. Any acute complication or sequela (including death) of an illness, disability, injury, or condition referred to above, which illness, disability, injury, or condition arose within the time period prescribed	Not applicable
IX. Hemophilus influenzae type b polysaccharide conjugate vaccines	No condition specified	Not applicable
X. Varicella vaccine	No condition specified	Not applicable
XI. Rotavirus vaccine	No condition specified	Not applicable
XII. Pneumococcal conjugate vaccines	No condition specified	Not applicable
XIII. Hepatitis A vaccines	No condition specified	Not applicable
XIV. Trivalent influenza vaccines	No condition specified	Not applicable
XV. Meningococcal vaccines	No condition specified	Not applicable

continued on page 129

XVI. Human papillomavirus (HPV) vaccines	No condition specified	Not applicable
XVII. Any new vaccine recommended by the Centers for Disease Control and Prevention for routine administration to children, after publication by the Secretary of a notice of coverage[d]	No condition specified	Not applicable

[a]Effective date: July 22, 2011.
[b]See qualifications and aids to interpretation of this table at www.hrsa.gov/vaccinecompensation/vaccinetable.html.
[c]Time period for first symptom or manifestation of onset or of significant aggravation after vaccine administration.
[d]Now includes all vaccines against seasonal influenza (except trivalent influenza vaccines, which are already covered), effective November 12, 2013.
Source: Reference 10.

Table 15.3

Emergency Supply Kit Contents

- Epinephrine (if using auto-injectors, at least three should be available)
- Diphenhydramine, if applicable
- Syringes and needles
- Alcohol swabs
- Blood pressure cuffs and stethoscope
- Wristwatch or clock with second hand
- CPR barrier or face shield
- Cold packs or compresses
- Sterile gauze or absorbent pads
- Medication dosing charts and record log

Table 15.4

Management of Adverse Vaccine Reactions

Adverse Reaction	Signs and Symptoms	Management Plan
Injection-site reaction	Soreness or erythema	• Apply a cold compress to the site for approximately 15 minutes. • May recommend an analgesic (i.e., acetaminophen) or nonsteroidal anti-inflammatory drug.
	Excessive bleeding[a]	• Apply firm pressure to the site using sterile gauze or absorbent pads. • Raise the arm above heart level.
	Itching and swelling	• Apply a cold compress to the site for approximately 15 minutes. • Recommend an antihistamine (e.g., diphenhydramine, chlorpheniramine). • Observe patient for generalized anaphylactic symptoms for at least 15 minutes. • Inform patient of signs and symptoms of anaphylaxis.
Syncope	Paleness, sweating, coldness of extremities, nausea, dizziness, weakness, visual disturbances, loss of consciousness	• If patient has fallen, check for injury. • Place patient in supine position with feet elevated. • Maintain an open airway. • Apply cold compresses to face, neck, and wrists. • Call 911 if patient does not immediately regain consciousness.

continued on page 131

Anaphylaxis	Generalized itching, erythema, urticaria (i.e., hives), angioedema, bronchospasm, shortness of breath, shock, abdominal cramping, cardiovascular collapse	• Instruct staff to call 911. • Place patient in supine position and maintain airway. • Assess airway, breathing, and circulation. • Administer epinephrine intramuscularly. • Consider administration of diphenhydramine as a secondary treatment option. • Perform CPR if necessary. • Repeat dose of epinephrine every 5 to 20 minutes, if needed, for up to three doses until EMS arrives.

[a]Bleeding may be more pronounced in patients taking antiplatelet or blood-thinning agents, such as aspirin or warfarin.
Adapted from: Reference 11.

Table 15.5

Epinephrine Dosing Based on Weight

Patient Weight	Intramuscular Dose
Epinephrine 1 mg/mL (1:1000 Dilution)	
4–8.5 kg (9–19 lb)	0.05 mg (0.05 mL)
9–14.5 kg (20–32 lb)	0.1 mg (0.1 mL)
15–17.5 kg (33–39 lb)	0.15 mg (0.15 mL)
18–25.5 kg (40–56 lb)	0.2–0.25 mg (0.2–0.25 mL)
26–34.5 kg (57–76 lb)	0.25–0.3 mg (0.25–0.3 mL)
35–45 kg (77–99 lb)	0.35–0.4 mg (0.35–0.4)
≥46 kg (≥100 lb)	0.5 mg (0.5 mL)
Epinephrine Auto-injector (Adrenaclick, Auvi-Q, EpiPen, EpiPen Jr., Twinject, generics)	
≤15 kg (≤ 33 lb)	Per the manufacturers' prescribing information, do not use auto-injector if ≤15 kg (≤ 33 lb). Use needle and syringe to withdraw correct dose from vial or ampul.
15–30 kg (33–66 lb)	0.15 mg
≥30 kg (≥66 lb)	0.3 mg

Adapted from: References 13, 16–20.

Table 15.6

Diphenhydramine Dosing Based on Weight

Patient Weight	Diphendyramine Dose (1–2 mg/kg every 4–6 hours)
9–14.5 kg (20–32 lb)	10–15 mg
15–17.5 kg (33–39 lb)	15–20 mg
18–25.5 kg (40–56 lb)	20–25 mg
26–45 kg (57–99 lb)	25–50 mg
≥46 kg (≥100 lb)	50 mg (up to a maximum of 100 mg per dose)

Adapted from: Reference 13.

Chapter 16

Recommendations for Immunocompromising and High-Risk Conditions

Some conditions or medications place patients at higher risk of contracting a vaccine-preventable disease or of experiencing more detrimental effects from the illness if they become infected. Many of these higher-risk patients will already be receiving care from a provider who specializes in treating their respective conditions, and immunizations will likely be a component of that care. Regardless, pharmacists may be presented with opportunities to educate and vaccinate these patients. This chapter summarizes recommendations for patients with commonly encountered high-risk or immunocompromising conditions. Pharmacists working with such patients will need to recognize when referral to a specialist is appropriate.

Altered Immunocompetence

Although certain vaccines are recommended for patients with altered immunocompetence because of these patients' increased risk of disease, the patients' state of immunosuppression may cause vaccines, particularly live, attenuated vaccines, to be less effective or more likely to result in an adverse reaction.[1] A patient's degree of altered immunocompetence should be determined by a physician or infectious disease specialist, as vaccine recommendations may depend on the level of immunosuppression.

Recommendations for vaccinating patients with altered immune systems vary by source. The Infectious Diseases Society of America (IDSA) published a new set of guidelines in 2013,[2] and some recommendations stemming from these guidelines differ from ACIP recommendations. Therefore, it is important to work with the patient and the patient's health care providers to determine the safest and most effective immunization options for that patient. Vaccine recommendations and differences by source are summarized in Table 16.1.[1–6] In the table, some routine adult vaccines may not have been included for some patients. If such omitted vaccines are indicated on the basis of other criteria for these patients and are not contraindicated, they may be used.

According to IDSA, patients can have either a low or a high level of immunosuppression (Table 16.2).[2] ACIP also categorizes patients with HIV infection on the basis of $CD4^+$ T-lymphocyte count, but it has not recognized the other situations defined by IDSA as low-level suppression to be problematic.[1]

As noted in Table 16.1, patients with immunocompromising conditions require both pneumococcal conjugate (PCV13) and pneumococcal polysaccharide (PPSV23) vaccines. The recommendations are specific to age group and whether or not patients have been previously vaccinated with one of the pneumococcal vaccines (Table 16.3).[5,6] For PCV13 to be fully effective, it needs to be given at least 8 weeks prior to PPSV23. If PPSV23 is given first, you must wait at least 1 year before administering PCV13.

Pregnancy and Breast-feeding

The vaccine recommendations for women who are pregnant or planning to become pregnant are intended to protect both the mother and her new baby. Live vaccines should be avoided during pregnancy because of the theoretical risk to the developing fetus. If live vaccines, in particular MMR and varicella, are indicated for a woman who is not yet pregnant, she should wait at least 28 days after vaccination to become pregnant. Otherwise, these vaccines should be administered immediately postpartum.

The inactivated influenza and Tdap vaccines are indicated during pregnancy. Pregnant women who get influenza are at much higher risk for complications from influenza, including death. Antibody transfer across the placenta provides protection for the newborn until the infant can be vaccinated.[1,8] Influenza and pertussis can be very detrimental to an infant, which is why the influenza and Tdap vaccines given to the pregnant patient are beneficial.

Pregnant patients may have other conditions that place them at high risk for additional vaccine-preventable illnesses. As long as these vaccines are not contraindicated, they may be recommended if the benefits of the vaccine outweigh the risks of the disease. Table 16.4 lists ACIP recommendations for pregnant patients.[9] Providers caring for pregnant patients who are planning international travel should consult *CDC Health Information for International Travel* (i.e., the Yellow Book) for additional guidance.

Questions often arise regarding the safety of vaccines for patients who are breast-feeding. The smallpox and yellow fever vaccines are the only two vaccines of concern. Smallpox is contraindicated, and yellow fever should be avoided unless travel places the woman at high risk. All other vaccines, both live and inactivated, are safe to administer to women who are breast-feeding.[1]

Other High-Risk Conditions

A variety of other conditions warrant specific immunizations to protect patients who are at high risk for infection or complications.[10–14] CDC's recommended adult immunization schedule provides guidance regarding vaccines that might be indicated for adults on the basis of medical and other conditions (www.cdc.gov/vaccines/schedules/downloads/adult/adult-combined-schedule.pdf). These CDC recommendations are summarized in Table 16.5.[10–14] The vaccines listed are those recommended because of the respective condition; other vaccines may be warranted per ACIP recommendations.

References

1. Centers for Disease Control and Prevention. General recommendations on immunization: recommendations of the Advisory Committee on Immunization Practices (ACIP). *MMWR Recomm Rep.* 2011;60(RR-2):1–64.
2. Rubin LG, Levin MJ, Ljungman P, et al. 2013 IDSA clinical practice guideline for vaccination of the immunocompromised host. *Clin Infect Dis.* 2014;58(3):e44–e100.
3. McCusker C, Warrington R. Primary immunodeficiency. *Allergy Asthma Clin Immunol.* 2011 Nov 10; 7 Suppl 1:S11. PMID: 22165913 [PubMed].
4. Centers for Disease Control and Prevention. Recommendations of the Advisory Committee on Immunization Practices (ACIP): use of vaccines and immune globulins in persons with altered immunocompetence. *MMWR Morbid Mortal Wkly Rep.* 1993;42(RR-4).
5. Centers for Disease Control and Prevention. Use of 13-valent pneumococcal conjugate vaccine and 23-valent pneumococcal polysaccharide vaccine for

adults with immunocompromising conditions: Recommendations of the Advisory Committee on Immunization Practices (ACIP). *MMWR Morb Mortal Wkly Rep.* 2012;61(40):816–9.
6. Centers for Disease Control and Prevention. Prevention of pneumococcal disease among infants and children—use of 13-valent pneumococcal conjugate vaccine and 23-valent pneumococcal polysaccharide vaccine. *MMWR Morb Mortal Wkly Rep.* 2010;59(RR-11):1–18.
7. Foster SL, Short CT, Angelo LB. Vaccination of patients with altered immunocompetence. *J Am Pharm Assoc.* 2013;53(4):438–40.
8. American College of Obstetricians and Gynecologists Immunization Expert Work Group, Committee on Obstetric Practice, and Committee on Gynecologic Practice. Integrating immunizations into practice. Committee Opinion No. 558, April 2013. *Obstet Gynecol.* 2013;121:897–903. www.acog.org/Resources-And-Publications/Committee-Opinions/Committee-on-Obstetric-Practice/Integrating-Immunizations-Into-Practice. Accessed October 14, 2014.
9. Centers for Disease Control and Prevention. Guidelines for vaccinating pregnant women. April 2013. www.cdc.gov/vaccines/pubs/downloads/b_preg_guide.pdf. Accessed October 15, 2014.
10. Immunization Action Coalition. Vaccinations for adults with diabetes. www.immunize.org/catg.d/p4043.pdf. Accessed October 14, 2014.
11. Immunization Action Coalition. Vaccinations for adults with heart disease. www.immunize.org/catg.d/p4044.pdf.
12. Immunization Action Coalition. Vaccinations for adults with hepatitis C infection. www.immunize.org/catg.d/p4042.pdf.
13. Immunization Action Coalition. Vaccinations for adults with lung disease. www.immunize.org/catg.d/p4045.pdf.
14. Centers for Disease Control and Prevention. Recommended adult immunization schedule—United States, 2014. www.cdc.gov/vaccines/schedules/downloads/adult/adult-combined-schedule.pdf. Accessed October 14, 2014.

Table 16.1

Vaccine Recommendations for Patients with Immunocompromising Conditions[a]

Contraindicated Vaccines	Recommended Vaccines	Comments
Asplenia		
Influenza (LAIV)[b]	Hib Influenza (inactivated) Meningococcal (MCV4) Pneumococcal (both PCV13 and PPSV23)	Revaccinate with meningococcal vaccine every 5 years.
Chemotherapy or Radiation Therapy[c]		
Influenza (LAIV) MMR Varicella Zoster	Hepatitis B Influenza (inactivated) Pneumococcal (both PCV13 and PPSV23) Td/Tdap	Vaccinate 2 weeks before starting therapy. Avoid vaccinating during therapy. If vaccines are given during therapy, patients may need to be revaccinated. Administer any necessary vaccines (including live vaccines) at least 3 months after therapy is complete and immune competence is regained. Td/Tdap is recommended for acute lymphoblastic leukemia and lymphoma.[b]
Chronic Kidney Disease		
Influenza (LAIV)	Hepatitis B Influenza (inactivated) Pneumococcal (both PCV13 and PPSV23)	

continued on page 138

Table 16.1

continued from page 137

Contraindicated Vaccines	Recommended Vaccines	Comments
Hematopoietic Stem Cell Transplant		
Influenza (LAIV) MMR Varicella Zoster	Hepatitis A Hepatitis B Hib Influenza (inactivated) Meningococcal (MCV4) Pneumococcal (both PCV13 and PPSV23) Polio (inactivated) Td/Tdap	Some live vaccines, if necessary, may be given if it has been at least 2 years since the transplant, no graft-versus-host disease (GVHD) is present, and the patient is not immunosuppressed.
HIV Infection (CD4$^+$ counts <200 cells/μL)[c]		
Influenza (LAIV) MMR Varicella Zoster	Hepatitis B HPV (if indicated) Influenza (inactivated) Pneumococcal (both PCV13 and PPSV23)	One dose of Hib may be given if necessary.
HIV Infection (CD4$^+$ ≥200 cells/μL)[c]		
Influenza (LAIV) MMRV[b] Zoster[b]	Hepatitis B HPV (if indicated) Influenza (inactivated) Pneumococcal (both PCV13 and PPSV23)	One dose of Hib may be given if appropriate.
Immune-Targeted Monoclonal Antibodies		
Safety and effectiveness of live vaccines unknown		Avoid administration of live vaccines until patient has regained immune competence.

continued on page 139

Solid Organ Transplant[c]		
Influenza (LAIV) MMR Varicella Zoster	Hepatitis A (liver transplant) Hepatitis B Influenza (inactivated) Pneumococcal (both PCV13 and PPSV23)	Avoid live vaccines after transplantation—vaccinate at least 2 weeks before transplantation.
Prolonged Systemic Corticosteroid Therapy[c,d]		
Influenza (LAIV) MMR Varicella Zoster	Influenza (inactivated) Pneumococcal (both PCV13 and PPSV23)	Wait 1 month after discontinuation of high-dose therapy before administering any live vaccines.

[a]Additional vaccines may be recommended on the basis of other risk factors.

[b]Per Infectious Diseases Society of America (IDSA) guidelines.

[c]The effectiveness of vaccines will vary depending on the degree of immunosuppression.

[d]Per IDSA guidelines, patients with low-level suppression due to medications (Table 16.2) age 50 and older should receive zoster but LAIV, MMR, and varicella are contraindicated; this differs from ACIP recommendations.

Source: References 1–6.

Table 16.2

IDSA Definitions of Immunosuppression

Low-Level Immunosuppression	High-Level Immunosuppression
$CD4^+$ counts ≥200 cells/μL	$CD4^+$ counts <200 cells/μL
Systemic corticosteroids equivalent to <2 mg/kg or <20 mg per day of prednisone for ≥14 days, or alternate-day therapy	Cancer chemotherapy
Methotrexate ≤0.4 mg/kg/day	Up to 2 months following solid organ transplant
Azathioprine ≤3 mg/kg/day	Immune-targeted monoclonal antibodies
Mercaptopurine ≤1.5 mg/kg/day	Systemic corticosteroids equivalent to ≥2 mg/kg or ≥20 mg per day of prednisone for ≥14 days
	Methotrexate >0.4 mg/kg/day
	Azathioprine >3 mg/kg/day
	Mercaptopurine >1.5 mg/kg/day

IDSA = Infectious Diseases Society of America.
Source: Reference 2.

Table 16.3

Pneumococcal Vaccine Recommendations for Immunocompromised Patients

Age Group	PCV13	PPSV23
≥24 months–71 months	If 3 doses of PCV7 were previously received, administer 1 dose of PCV13. If fewer than 3 doses of PCV7 were previously received, administer 2 doses of PCV13 at least 8 weeks apart.	Administer 1 dose at least 8 weeks after last PCV13 dose. Revaccinate with 1 dose 5 years after the first PPSV23 dose.
≥6–18 years	If not previously vaccinated with PCV13, administer 1 dose.	If not previously vaccinated with PPSV23, administer 1 dose at least 8 weeks after last PCV13 dose. Revaccinate with 1 dose 5 years after the first PPSV23 dose.
≥19 years, not previously vaccinated with PPSV23	Administer 1 dose of PCV13 as soon as possible.	Administer 1 dose at least 8 weeks after PCV13 dose. Revaccinate after 5 years and again at ≥65 years if 5 years have passed since last dose.
≥19 years, previously vaccinated with PPSV23	Administer 1 dose of PCV13 at least 1 year after last PPSV23 dose.	If it has been 5 years since last PPSV23 dose and an additional dose is required, wait at least 8 weeks after PCV13 dose.

Source: Reprinted with permission from reference 7.

Table 16.4

Vaccine Recommendations for Pregnant Patients

Recommended

- Influenza (inactivated)—Vaccinate in any trimester during influenza season
- Tdap—Administer a dose during each pregnancy, ideally between 27 and 36 weeks of gestation

Recommended if Another Risk Factor Is Present

- Hepatitis A
- Hepatitis B
- Meningococcal conjugate (MCV4)
- Pneumococcal polysaccharide (PPSV23)
- Polio (inactivated)

Not Recommended

- Human papillomavirus

Contraindicated

- Influenza (LAIV)
- MMR
- Varicella
- Zoster

Source: Reference 9.

Table 16.5

Vaccine Recommendations for Adults with Commonly Encountered High-Risk Conditions

Condition	Recommended Vaccine(s)[a]
Diabetes	Hepatitis B Influenza (inactivated) Pneumococcal polysaccharide (PPSV23)
Heart disease	Influenza (inactivated) Pneumococcal polysaccharide (PPSV23)
Hepatitis C	Hepatitis A Hepatitis B Influenza (inactivated) Pneumococcal polysaccharide (PPSV23)
Lung disease	Influenza (inactivated) Pneumococcal polysaccharide (PPSV23)
Smoking	Influenza (LAIV, if not otherwise contraindicated, or inactivated) Pneumococcal polysaccharide (PPSV23)

[a]It is recommended that all adults get the influenza and Tdap vaccines, regardless of medical condition.

Source: References 10–14.

Chapter 17

Infection Control in the Pharmacy Setting

First and foremost, pharmacists and pharmacy personnel involved in immunization activities need to protect themselves from infection and illness. If you or your staff become ill, especially with a communicable disease, the care you are able to provide to your patients may be compromised. You may miss work. Worse yet, if you go to work sick, you are putting your patients at risk for infection. Since your job responsibilities and the environment in which you work place you at risk of acquiring and transmitting infections,[1] you must take responsibility for infection control.

Vaccines for Health Care Personnel

You and your staff should be immunized against the vaccine-preventable diseases for which you are most at risk, as well as those that place your patients at risk should you become ill. In fact, the 2011 APhA House of Delegates adopted a policy supporting the requirement of annual influenza vaccination for all eligible individuals who provide pharmacy-related services.[2] Numerous other professional associations have adopted similar policies endorsing mandatory influenza vaccination of health care personnel.[3] Health systems nationwide have begun to require annual influenza vaccination for all employees. If vaccination is declined, employees will be asked to take other preventive measures, such as wearing medical face masks.[4–6] Having 90% of health care personnel vaccinated against seasonal influenza is a Healthy People 2020 target.[7] In addition to influenza, several other vaccines are currently recommended for health care personnel (Table 17.1).[8–10] Additional vaccines may be recommended for health care personnel if specific circumstances place them at risk for infection.[8]

OSHA and the Bloodborne Pathogens Standard

Exposure to bloodborne pathogens (BBPs) presents another inherent risk for infection. The pathogens of concern are hepatitis B virus (HBV), hepatitis C virus (HCV), and human immunodeficiency virus (HIV). Contact with an infected patient's blood or bodily fluids via needlesticks or cuts from other sharp objects presents an exposure risk. If you are administering a vaccine or disposing of sharps and biohazardous waste, you are at risk for BBP exposure. All employees whose job functions put them at risk for exposure must receive annual training in compliance with the OSHA Bloodborne Pathogens Standard. Education regarding BBPs and the mechanisms by which exposures occur is important for preventing occupational contact with blood and other potentially infectious material.[11] It is the responsibility of the employer to provide this training. Table 17.2 lists training and educational resources available from OSHA. Numerous companies and organizations offer OSHA BBP training (e.g., medical waste disposal companies, APhA and other professional pharmacy associations, *Pharmacist's Letter,* the American Red Cross). If you outsource a training program, you will need to customize or add to the information to fit the needs of your employees and the risks inherent to your practice. As an employer, you have the option of creating your own training program so long as it is developed and taught by knowledgeable individuals and includes the training components required by OSHA. At-risk employees should also be offered the HBV vaccine at no cost. If they initially decline the vaccine, they should have the option to request the vaccine later. Their acceptance or refusal of the vaccine must be documented. The OSHA-mandated documentation requirements are detailed in Chapter 8.

OSHA compliance checklist for providers of pharmacy-based immunization programs[12,13]

- ☐ Read the OSHA Bloodborne Pathogens Standard (29 CFR 1910.1030), which can be accessed via the OSHA website (www.osha.gov/law-regs.html).
- ☐ Provide annual OSHA training to all employees with exposure risk, and document the provision of such training.
- ☐ Offer HBV vaccine to all employees with exposure risk, and document their receipt or refusal of the vaccine.
- ☐ Develop an exposure control plan, which must be reviewed and updated annually.
- ☐ Require employees to observe universal precautions, whereby all blood and bodily fluids are considered infectious.
- ☐ Incorporate engineering and work practice controls (e.g., sharps disposal containers, safer medical devices, prohibition of needle recapping).

continued on page 147

OSHA compliance checklist, *continued from page 146*

- ☐ Provide employees with personal protective equipment (i.e., disposable gloves, laboratory coats, CPR barriers or face shields).
- ☐ Review, select, and annually evaluate sharps (i.e., needles) with engineered sharps injury protection. Employee input should be used during this evaluation and selection process.
- ☐ Create and maintain a sharps injury log.
- ☐ Maintain medical records for all employees with occupational exposure for the duration of employment plus 30 years.

According to OSHA, 27 states and jurisdictions have developed their own occupational safety and health plans, which have been approved by OSHA.[14] Many states have additional safeguards and requirements, including needle safety legislation.[15] To determine the complete scope of regulations applicable in your state, you will need to consult your state and local regulatory agencies.

Tips for avoiding OSHA citations[13]

- Have your exposure control plan (ECP) accessible at all times in all locations where vaccines are given.
- Review and update your ECP annually.
- Review and implement commercially available "safer medical devices."
- Implement procedures for documenting exposure incidents.
- Follow universal precautions.
- Comply with current recommendations from CDC for postexposure evaluation and follow-up.
- Never recap used needles.
- Do not dispose of needle caps in the sharps disposal container. Needles could be inadvertently recapped when dropped into a container containing caps.

Needlestick Prevention

The needles and syringes used for immunizations should come equipped with safety features or mechanisms to minimize the risk of needlesticks and BBP exposure. All employees who will be using the devices should be given the opportunity to evaluate a variety of commercially available syringes and needles with safety features and to provide feedback on whether they should be used. This should be done annually. Figure 17.1 shows a sample form for collecting employee feedback.

Needlestick prevention tips

- Practice the process of needle insertion, withdrawal, safety device activation, and disposal until you are comfortable before administering a vaccine to a patient. An injection pad or an orange can be used for practice.
- Administer vaccines in an area with minimal distractions.
- Stabilize your patient at all times.
- Do not administer vaccines to a patient who appears agitated or restless.
- Watch the needle at all times, from the moment it enters the patient until it is dropped into the sharps disposal container.
- Know how to activate the safety device before you administer a vaccine to a patient.
- Dispose of the needle before providing injection site care.
- Keep the sharps disposal container within arm's reach so that you do not reach across your own body or the patient's to dispose of the needle.
- Never recap a used needle.
- Never reach into a sharps disposal container.

Exposure Control Plan

OSHA requires that employers establish a written exposure control plan (ECP) with the intent of minimizing or preventing their employees' exposure risk.[12] The ECP must include the following elements:

- Determination of employee exposure, listing job classifications and responsibilities in which exposure may occur
- Implementation and control methods for the ECP, including but not limited to the following:
    - Universal precautions
    - ECP education for employees
    - ECP availability, review, and revision processes
    - Engineering and work practice controls
    - Personal protective equipment

    - Housekeeping
    - Laundry
    - Labels
- Hepatitis B vaccination for employees
- Postexposure evaluation and follow-up
- Administration of postexposure evaluation and follow-up
- Procedures for evaluating the circumstances surrounding an exposure incident
- Employee training
- Record keeping for training records, medical records, OSHA, and sharps injury log
- Hepatitis B vaccine declination (refusal) statement

A sample ECP can be found at www.osha.gov/Publications/osha3186.pdf.

Your ECP should be specific to your practice site and should address the expected tasks of your employees. It must be accessible to your employees at all times. The plan should be reviewed and updated at least annually or whenever changes occur that affect occupational exposure at your site. In developing and updating the plan, the input of nonmanagerial employees should be solicited.

Hand Hygiene

One of the simplest, and perhaps most important, measures for infection control in the pharmacy environment is the practice of hand hygiene. This applies to both health care personnel and patients. Poor adherence to hand hygiene policies has been linked to increased infections and outbreaks in the health care arena.[16] Engineering and work practice controls should include adherence measures for hand hygiene. The Bloodborne Pathogens Standard states that hand washing facilities must be readily accessible to employees. When the provision of such facilities is not feasible, either an antiseptic hand cleanser and towels (paper or cloth) or antiseptic towelettes should be provided, after which the hands should be washed with soap and running water as soon as feasible.[12] Personnel should use hand hygiene measures whenever they come into contact with a patient's skin or environmental surfaces in the vicinity of patients, and upon glove removal.[16] Wearing gloves does not replace the need for hand hygiene. To ensure compliance with hand hygiene practices, patients and providers must have easy access to supplies (e.g., running water and soap or medicated detergent, alcohol-based hand sanitizer). These should be readily available in the pharmacy and in locations where vaccines are given. Place hand sanitizer for patients to use in locations where surface contact is high (e.g., waiting areas, prescription drop-off window, prescription pickup or payment window). Patients may also appreciate access to hand sanitizers after they are required to use shared pens or the devices used to sign electronic signature logs.

Infection Control Measures during Disease Outbreaks

When an outbreak occurs, there is a heightened level of awareness about disease transmission and infection control. This is especially true in health care facilities, where health care personnel must be protected from ill patients and patients must be protected from ill staff members and other patients. Certain measures can be taken to reduce exposure to and spread of disease. If a vaccine is available for the disease of concern, health care personnel should be encouraged, and in some instances required, to be vaccinated. In fact, during the 2009 H1N1 influenza pandemic, health care personnel were among the priority groups to receive the 2009 H1N1 influenza vaccine. It was provided free of charge, and employers were encouraged to offer the vaccine during working hours.[17] Vaccination was considered one of the most important interventions to keep health care providers from contracting the influenza virus. Additional measures that pharmacists and employers can take during an outbreak or pandemic include the following:[17–19]

- Identify health care professionals and staff who are at increased risk for complications if they become ill, so that vaccination and early treatment can be provided.
- Provide written guidance for employees on the actions they need to take if they become ill.
- Create sick leave policies that are flexible, nonpunitive, and consistent with public health guidance to allow pharmacists and staff who are ill to stay at home.
- Develop a contingency plan for potential staff shortages due to illness.
- Consider providing chemoprophylaxis for employees when available and warranted.

- Educate pharmacists and staff about the signs and symptoms of the disease, patient education strategies, and employee policies.
- Post signs around the pharmacy instructing patients to notify staff if they have signs and symptoms of the disease, so that precautions can be taken.
- For diseases transmitted by respiratory droplets, enforce respiratory hygiene and cough etiquette.
- For diseases transmitted by respiratory droplets, provide face masks for both patients and employees. (Although face masks may not filter small particles from the air, they can serve as physical barriers to droplet sprays as well as hand to nose and mouth autoinoculation of the virus.)
- Place tissues, touch-free disposal receptacles, and hand sanitizer around the pharmacy counter and in the waiting areas.
- Install temporary partitions around the pharmacy and in the waiting area.
- Arrange seating and waiting areas to allow ample space between patients.

Infection Control—A Personal Responsibility

Each pharmacy staff person must assume personal responsibility for infection control. Infection control education and written policies and procedures are key.[1] Health care personnel who understand the consequences of infections, the reasons for preventing them, and how to apply infection control procedures will be instrumental in reducing the occurrence and transmission of communicable disease.

References

1. Centers for Disease Control and Prevention. Guideline for infection control in health care personnel, 1998. www.cdc.gov/hicpac/pdf/InfectControl98.pdf. Accessed October 12, 2014.

2. American Pharmacists Association. Report of the 2011 APhA House of Delegates. *J Am Pharm Assoc.* 2011;51(4):482–4.

3. Immunization Action Coalition. Honor roll for patient safety. http://www.immunize.org/honor-roll/. Accessed October 12, 2014.

4. Ho V. Mandatory flu shots or your job? Hospitals get tough with workers. *Seattlepi.com.* November 14, 2010. www.seattlepi.com/default/article/Mandatory-flu-shots-or-your-job-Hospitals-get-813091.php. Accessed October 12, 2014.

5. Hospital of Saint Raphael. Saint Raphael's flu vaccination policy promotes prevention. *Connecticutplus.com.* February 1, 2011. www.connecticutplus.com/cplus/information/news/health/Saint-Raphael-s-flu-vaccination-policy-promotes-prevention1159311593.shtml. Accessed October 12, 2014.
6. Washington State Hospital Association. Reduce hospital acquired infections: healthcare worker influenza immunization. www.wsha.org/files/82/FluSupport.docx. Accessed October 12, 2014.
7. U.S. Department of Health and Human Services. Healthy People 2020 topics & objectives: immunization and infectious diseases. www.healthypeople.gov/2020/topics-objectives/topic/immunization-and-infectious-diseases/objectives. Accessed October 12, 2014.
8. Centers for Disease Control and Prevention. Immunization of health-care personnel: recommendations of the Advisory Committee on Immunization Practices (ACIP). *MMWR Recomm Rep.* 2011;60(RR-07):1–45.
9. Centers for Disease Control and Prevention. Recommended adult immunization schedule—United States, 2014. www.cdc.gov/vaccines/schedules/downloads/adult/adult-pocket-size.pdf. Accessed October 12, 2014.
10. Immunization Action Coalition. Healthcare personnel vaccination recommendations. www.immunize.org/catg.d/p2017.pdf. Accessed October 12, 2014.
11. Cardo DM, Bell DM. Bloodborne pathogen transmission in health care workers: risks and prevention strategies. *Infect Dis Clin North Am.* 1997;11(2):331–46.
12. Bloodborne pathogens. 29 CFR 1910.1030 (2010). www.osha.gov/pls/oshaweb/owadisp.show_document?p_table=STANDARDS&p_id=10051. Accessed October 12, 2014.
13. American Pharmacists Association. Pharmacy-Based Immunization Delivery: A National Certificate Program for Pharmacists. 11th ed. Washington, DC: American Pharmacists Association; 2009.
14. U.S. Department of Labor, Occupational Safety and Health Administration. Frequently asked questions about state occupational safety and health plans. www.osha.gov/dcsp/osp/faq.html#N_2. Accessed October 12, 2014.
15. Centers for Disease Control and Prevention, National Institute for Occupational Safety and Health. State-by-state provisions of state needle safety regulation (revised June 2002) in chronological order. www.cdc.gov/niosh/topics/bbp/ndl-law-1.html. Accessed October 12, 2014.
16. Centers for Disease Control and Prevention. Guideline for hand hygiene in health-care settings: recommendations of the Healthcare Infection Control Practices Advisory Committee and the HICPAC/SHEA/APIC/IDSA Hand Hygiene Task Force. *MMWR Recomm Rep.* 2002;51(RR-16). www.cdc.gov/mmwr/PDF/rr/rr5116.pdf. Accessed October 12, 2014.

17. Centers for Disease Control and Prevention. Interim guidance on infection control measures for 2009 H1N1 influenza in healthcare settings, including protection of healthcare personnel. July 15, 2010. www.cdc.gov/h1n1flu/guidelines_infection_control.htm. Accessed October 12, 2014.
18. Centers for Disease Control and Prevention. Prevention strategies for seasonal influenza in healthcare settings. www.cdc.gov/flu/professionals/infectioncontrol/healthcaresettings.htm. Accessed October 12, 2014.
19. Centers for Disease Control and Prevention. Guide to infection prevention for outpatient settings: minimum expectations for safe care. www.cdc.gov/HAI/settings/outpatient/outpatient-care-guidelines.html. Accessed October 12, 2014.

Table 17.1

Vaccines Routinely Recommended for Health Care Personnel (HCP)

Vaccine	Recommendations
Hepatitis B	For HCP whose job responsibilities involve potential exposure to blood or bodily fluids; perform serologic testing for antibody to hepatitis B surface antigen (anti-HBs) 1 to 2 months after third dose
Influenza	Administer annually
Measles, mumps, rubella (MMR)[a]	Two doses are recommended for HCP born during or after 1957 without serologic evidence of immunity or prior vaccination; consider two doses for unvaccinated HCP born before 1957 who do not have laboratory-confirmed evidence of disease or immunity
Varicella[a]	Recommended unless evidence of immunity exists
Tetanus, diphtheria, pertussis	Substitute one-time dose of Td with Tdap for HCP regardless of age, even if <10 years since last Td; administer to pregnant women preferably during 27–36 weeks' gestation; Td booster every 10 years

[a]Contraindicated in pregnant patients, patients with immunocompromising conditions, and those with HIV who have CD4$^+$ T-lymphocyte count <200 cells/μL.

Source: References: 8–10.

Table 17.2

OSHA Training and Educational Resources for Pharmacy Employers and Employees

Resource Type	Source, Title, and Location
Training components and requirements	Occupational Safety and Health Administration—29 CFR 1910.1030(q)(2); www.osha.gov/SLTC/bloodborne pathogens/index.html; click the Standards tab and go to 1910.1030(g)(2)
Brochure for employees	Centers for Disease Control and Prevention; Exposure to Blood: What Healthcare Personnel Need to Know; www.cdc.gov/HAI/pdfs/bbp/Exp_to_Blood.pdf
OSHA's blood-borne pathogens PowerPoint presentation	Occupational Safety and Health Administration; OSHA's Revised Bloodborne Pathogens Standard; www.osha.gov/dte/library/bloodborne/revised_bbp_standard/index.html
Compliance information and resources for employers	National Institute for Occupational Safety and Health; Information for Employers: Complying with OSHA's Bloodborne Pathogens Standard; www.cdc.gov/niosh/docs/2009-111/
Sharps injury protection workbook	Centers for Disease Control and Prevention; Workbook for Designing, Implementing, and Evaluating a Sharps Injury Prevention Program; www.cdc.gov/sharpssafety/resources.html
List of safety devices	University of Virginia Health System—Safety Device List; www.healthsystem.virginia.edu/pub/epinet/new/safetydevice.html
Preventing needlestick injuries	National Institute for Occupational Safety and Health; NIOSH Alert: Preventing Needlestick Injuries in Health Care Settings; www.cdc.gov/niosh/docs/2000-108/
Exposure control plan elements and improvement tips	National Institute for Occupational Safety and Health; Protect Your Employees with an Exposure Control Plan; www.cdc.gov/niosh/docs/2008-115/pdfs/2008-115.pdf

Figure 17.1

Sample Form for Evaluating Sharps with Engineered Sharps Injury Protection (SESIP).[a]

All employees involved with immunizations should be given the opportunity to evaluate a variety of commercially available devices (i.e., syringes and needles) with safety features. Upon evaluation, each employee should complete this form. The devices with the overall highest scores should be the ones available for employee use when administering vaccines.

Name of device: ____

Manufacturer: ____

What type of safety feature does this device have?

☐ Self-sheathing ☐ Retractable technology ☐ Hinge device

Is this device available in the sizes and/or gauges that are most applicable to your practice site and patient care activities?

☐ Yes ☐ No

If you answered "no" to this question, do not order this device.

Rank your extent of agreement with the following statements regarding features of the device:

(1=Strongly Disagree, 5 = Strongly Agree)

	1	2	3	4	5
The device is easy to use.	☐	☐	☐	☐	☐
The safety feature is simple to operate.	☐	☐	☐	☐	☐
I am comfortable with the degree of safety the device offers.	☐	☐	☐	☐	☐
The time it takes to activate the safety mechanism is minimal.	☐	☐	☐	☐	☐
There is a very low risk of error when using the device.	☐	☐	☐	☐	☐
I can activate the safety mechanism with one hand.	☐	☐	☐	☐	☐
I can either hear or see when the safety feature has been activated.	☐	☐	☐	☐	☐
The device does not inflict additional pain or discomfort on the patient.	☐	☐	☐	☐	☐
I did not need extensive training to learn how to use the device.	☐	☐	☐	☐	☐
The quantity and type of sharps disposal containers will not change as a result of this device.	☐	☐	☐	☐	☐
The device is readily available from wholesalers or distributors.	☐	☐	☐	☐	☐
The device is affordable.	☐	☐	☐	☐	☐
Column totals					

Total device score: ________

Additional comments:

[a]*A needle with a built-in safety feature or mechanism that reduces risk of exposure.*

Immunization and Vaccine Product Information

Chapter 18

Frequently Asked Questions about Immunizations

Because this book is intended as a concise handbook, the preceding chapters have addressed some topics only briefly or not at all. This chapter, which provides answers to some questions that often arise about vaccines, supplements the content of the previous chapters. The information has been extracted in part from the "Ask the Experts" forum provided by the Immunization Action Coalition (IAC) (www.immunize.org/askexperts). IAC has granted permission for use of its information. IAC's experts are affiliated with the Centers for Disease Control and Prevention (CDC); they include medical officer Andrew T. Kroger, MD, MPH, and nurse educator Donna L. Weaver, RN, MN, at the National Center for Immunization and Respiratory Diseases, CDC. William L. Atkinson, MD, MPH, is acknowledged for his contributions to updating the content in this chapter.

The topics addressed in this chapter include the following:

Influenza

Is it acceptable to administer a dose of the quadrivalent influenza vaccine to a patient who has already received the trivalent vaccine?
No. ACIP does not recommend that anyone receive more than one dose of influenza vaccine in a season, except for certain children age 6 months through 8 years for whom two doses are recommended.

If a patient received a dose of influenza vaccine in June (for example, for international travel), how long should the patient wait before getting vaccinated with the next season's flu vaccine?
There should be a minimum of 4 weeks between the doses in such situations.

Why do people who received influenza vaccine in one year still need to get vaccinated in the next year when the viruses haven't changed?
It is true that the strains may sometimes be the same as in the previous year's vaccine, but the antibody titers that persons might have achieved from the previous year's vaccination will have waned and will need to be boosted with a dose of the current year's vaccine. You should *not* use the previous season's vaccine that you might still have in your refrigerator. Most influenza vaccine distributed in the northern hemisphere expires on June 30 after each season; expired vaccine should *never* be administered.

Sometimes patients age 65 years and older who have received the standard-dose influenza vaccine hear about the high-dose product (Sanofi's Fluzone High-Dose) and want to receive that, too. Is this okay to administer?
No. ACIP does not recommend that anyone receive more than one dose of influenza vaccine in a season, except for certain children age 6 months through 8 years for whom two doses are recommended.

What is the latest ACIP guidance on influenza vaccination and egg allergy?
People who have experienced a serious systemic or anaphylactic reaction (for example, hives, swelling of the lips or tongue, acute respiratory distress, or collapse) after eating eggs should consult a specialist for appropriate evaluation to help determine whether vaccine should be administered. A previous severe allergic reaction to influenza vaccine, regardless of the component suspected to be responsible for the reaction, is a contraindication to future receipt of the vaccine.

People who have documented immunoglobulin E (IgE)-mediated hypersensitivity to eggs, including those who have had occupational asthma or other allergic responses to egg protein, might also be at increased risk for allergic reactions to influenza vaccine. Protocols have been published for safely administering egg-based influenza vaccine to people with egg allergies. Some people who report allergy to egg might not be egg allergic. A person who can eat lightly cooked eggs (for example, scrambled eggs) is unlikely to have an egg allergy. However, people who can tolerate egg in baked products (for example, cake) might still have an egg allergy. If the person develops hives only after ingesting eggs, CDC recommends that (1) the person receive IIV (not LAIV), (2) the vaccine be administered by a health care provider familiar with the potential manifestations of egg allergy, and (3) the vaccine recipient be observed for at least 30 minutes after receipt of the vaccine for signs of a reaction. An inactivated influenza vaccine that does not contain egg protein is now available in the United States.

If an unvaccinated patient who has just recovered from a diagnosed case of influenza comes into our clinic, should we vaccinate him?

Yes. The trivalent influenza vaccine contains three influenza vaccine virus strains, two for A viruses and one for a B virus; quadrivalent influenza vaccine contains two A strains and two B strains. These vaccines are formulated on the basis of circulating viruses from the previous influenza season. Infection by one virus type does not confer immunity to other types, and it is not unusual to have exposure to more than one type during a typical influenza season. By all means, vaccinate this person!

Some of my patients refuse influenza vaccination because they insist they "got the flu" after receiving the injectable vaccine in the past. What can I tell them?

There are several reasons why this misconception persists: (1) Fewer than 1% of people who are vaccinated with the injectable vaccine develop flu-like symptoms, such as mild fever and muscle aches, after vaccination. These side effects are not the same as having influenza, but people confuse the symptoms. (2) Protective immunity does not develop until 1 to 2 weeks after vaccination. Some people who are vaccinated later in the season (December or later) may get influenza shortly afterward. These late vaccinees develop influenza because they were exposed to someone with the virus before they became immune. It is not the result of the vaccination. (3) To many people, "the flu" is any illness with fever and cold symptoms. If they get any viral illness, they may blame it on the flu shot or think they got "the flu" despite being vaccinated. Influenza vaccine protects only against certain influenza viruses, not all viruses. (4) The influenza vaccine is not 100% effective, especially in older persons. The vaccine is effective in protecting 90% of healthy young adult vaccinees from illness when the vaccine strain is similar to the circulating strain. However, the vaccine is only 30%–40% effective in preventing illness among frail elderly persons (although among elderly persons, the vaccine is 50%–60% effective in preventing hospitalization and 80% effective in preventing death).

Can live attenuated influenza virus (LAIV) be administered to persons with minor acute illnesses, such as a mild upper respiratory infection (URI) with or without fever?

Yes. However, if clinical judgment suggests nasal congestion that is present might impede delivery of the vaccine to the nasopharyngeal mucosa, you should consider deferring administration until the congestion resolves or administer an inactivated influenza vaccine.

Hepatitis A

Why is hepatitis A vaccination recommended for people with chronic liver disease?

Although not at increased risk for hepatitis A virus (HAV) infection, people with chronic liver disease are at increased risk for fulminant hepatitis A if they should become infected with HAV. For this reason, hepatitis A vaccination is recommended for them.

Why does a 15-year old who weighs 160 pounds receive a pediatric dose of hepatitis A vaccine while his 110-pound mother receives an adult dose (twice the pediatric dose)?

The efficacy data from the clinical trials were based on age at the time of vaccination, not on the weight of the individual. Hence, the dosage recommendations reflect this age-based efficacy data. The same holds true for hepatitis B vaccine. In addition, higher response rates are expected in younger people, even if their weights are above the norm.

Hepatitis B

How stable is the hepatitis B virus (HBV) in the environment, and what types of equipment cleaners are virucidal against HBV?

Any high-level disinfectant that is tuberculocidal will kill HBV. It is important to note that HBV is quite stable in the environment and remains viable for 7 or more days on environmental surfaces at room temperature. The virus can still be transmitted despite the absence of visible blood.

Is postvaccination testing needed for adults who receive hepatitis B vaccine?

Serologic testing for immunity after vaccination is recommended only for persons whose subsequent clinical management depends on knowledge of their immune status. Testing is not necessary after routine vaccination of adults.

Postvaccination testing is recommended for the following: health care and public safety workers at high risk of continued exposure to blood on the job, immunocompromised persons, and sex or needle-sharing partners of hepatitis B surface antigen (HBsAg)-positive persons. Testing should be performed 1 to 2 months after the last dose of vaccine.

What should be done if a health care worker's serologic test comes back negative for anti-HBs (antibody to HBsAg) 1 to 2 months after the last dose of vaccine?

Repeat the three-dose series and test for anti-HBs 1 to 2 months after the last dose of vaccine. If the worker still tests negative after a second vaccine series, he or she is considered a nonresponder to hepatitis B vaccination. Health care workers who do not respond to vaccination should be tested for HBsAg to determine if they have chronic HBV infection. If the HBsAg test is positive, the person should receive appropriate counseling and medical management. Persons who test negative for HBsAg should be considered susceptible to HBV infection and should be counseled about precautions to prevent HBV infection and the need to obtain hepatitis B immune globulin (HBIG) prophylaxis for any known or likely parenteral exposure to HBsAg-positive blood.

How should vaccinated health care workers with an unknown anti-HBs response be managed if they have a percutaneous or mucosal exposure to blood or body fluids from an HBsAg-positive source?

These persons should be tested for anti-HBs as soon as possible after exposure. If the anti-HBs concentration is at least 10 mIU/mL, no further treatment is needed. If the anti-HBs concentration is less than 10 mIU/mL,

HBIG and hepatitis B vaccine should be administered. In addition, the person should receive postvaccination anti-HBs testing in 3 to 6 months. It is necessary to do postvaccination testing later than the usual recommended time frame of 1 to 2 months because anti-HBs from HBIG might be detected if testing were done earlier. The postvaccination test result should be recorded in the person's health record.

How long should a person wait to donate blood or have an HBsAg blood test after a dose of hepatitis B vaccine?

It is advisable to wait 1 month. Studies published in the past several years have found that transient HBsAg-positivity (lasting less than 21 days) can be detected in certain people after vaccination. This does not mean the person is infected with HBV. However, donating too close to receipt of hepatitis B vaccine could cause a person to be permanently deferred from blood donation if that person tests transiently HBsAg positive after the vaccine dose.

Does the recommendation to administer hepatitis B vaccine to persons younger than age 60 with diabetes extend to women with gestational diabetes?

No. The 2011 CDC recommendations for hepatitis B vaccination of people with diabetes pertain to those with type 1 and type 2 diabetes. They do not apply to women with gestational diabetes. Women with type 1 or type 2 diabetes who become pregnant can be vaccinated, if indicated, since pregnancy is not a contraindication to hepatitis B vaccination. These recommendations can be found in the December 23, 2011, issue of *Morbidity and Mortality Weekly Report.*

We've heard that there is an alternative schedule for the adult hepatitis A–hepatitis B vaccine (Twinrix; GlaxoSmithKline) that gives the patient protection sooner than the standard schedule does. Can you tell us more?

Licensed for use in people age 18 and older, the combined hepatitis A–hepatitis B vaccine is normally given as a three-dose series at intervals of 0, 1, and 6 months. However, if someone needs protection sooner (e.g., for imminent foreign travel), you can give it as a four-dose series at intervals of 0, 7, and 21–30 days followed by a dose at 12 months.

Haemophilus influenzae type b (Hib)

Which adults should receive Hib vaccine?

Hib vaccine is not routinely recommended for healthy adults 19 years and older, even if the person did not receive Hib vaccine as a child. However, ACIP recommends that Hib vaccine can be administered to persons with anatomic or functional asplenia if they have not previously received Hib vaccine. One standard pediatric dose of any Hib vaccine may be used. Regardless of Hib vaccination history, recipients of hematopoietic stem cell transplants should receive three doses of Hib vaccine at least 4 weeks apart beginning 6–12 months after transplant.

When should Hib vaccine be administered to a person having a splenectomy?

When elective splenectomy is planned, vaccination with pneumococcal, meningococcal, and Hib vaccines should precede surgery by at least 2 weeks, if possible. If vaccines are not administered before surgery, they should be administered as soon as the person's condition stabilizes postoperatively.

Human Papillomavirus (HPV)

Is it recommended that patients age 26 years start the HPV vaccination series even though they will be older than 26 when they complete it?

Yes. HPV vaccine is recommended for all women through age 26 years and also may be given to men through that age. So, the three-dose series can be started at age 26 even if it will not be completed at age 26. The series should be completed regardless of the age of the patient (i.e., even if the patient is older than 26). In certain situations, some clinicians choose to start the three-dose HPV series in patients who are older than 26 years. This, however, is an off-label use.

If a 30-year-old female patient insists that she wants to be given HPV vaccine, can I give it to her?

HPV vaccine currently is not FDA-licensed for use in women older than age 26 years. ACIP does not recommend the use of this vaccine outside the FDA licensing guidelines; however, physicians may administer this vaccine off-label. There is no reason to believe the vaccine would be any less safe for women in this age group than for younger women. Clinicians should decide whether the benefit of the vaccine outweighs the hypothetical risk.

If a woman is diagnosed with HPV infection, should she still be vaccinated?
Yes. Although the vaccine would not alter the clinical course of the current infection, the woman would still benefit from protection against the other virus types in the vaccine.

Meningococcal

What is the difference between the two meningococcal vaccines, MPSV and MCV?
Meningococcal conjugate vaccine (MCV), licensed in 2005, is believed to have several advantages over meningococcal polysaccharide vaccine (MPSV), such as reduction in bacterial carriage in the nose and throat, longer duration of immunity, and better immunologic memory. These advantages may result in better herd immunity.

I've heard that the recently updated recommendations for use of meningococcal conjugate vaccines in adolescents now include a booster dose. Would you please tell me more?
ACIP recommends that children age 11 or 12 years be routinely vaccinated with quadrivalent meningococcal conjugate vaccine (MCV4) and receive a booster dose at age 16. Adolescents who receive the first dose at age 13–15 should receive a one-time booster dose, preferably at age 16–18, the years before the peak in occurrence of meningococcal disease. Teens who receive their first dose of meningococcal conjugate vaccine at or after age 16 do not need a booster dose, as long as they have no risk factors.

Which previously vaccinated college students need a booster dose of MCV4?
A booster dose should be given to first-year college students age 21 years and younger who are or will be living in a residence hall if the previous dose was given before the age of 16 years.

Measles, Mumps, and Rubella Virus Vaccine (MMR)

If a health care worker develops a rash and low-grade fever after MMR vaccine, is the worker infectious?

Approximately 5%–15% of susceptible people who receive MMR vaccine will develop a low-grade fever, a mild rash, or both 7–12 days after vaccination. However, these persons are not infectious, and no special precautions (e.g., exclusion from work) need to be taken.

Can I give a tuberculin skin test (TST) on the same day as a dose of MMR vaccine?

A TST can be applied before or on the same day that MMR vaccine is given. However, if MMR vaccine is given on the previous day or earlier, the TST should be delayed for at least 1 month. Administration of live measles vaccine before the application of a TST can reduce the reactivity of the skin test because of mild suppression of the immune system.

Pneumococcal

Which children should receive PPSV23 vaccine (in addition to PCV13)? At what age should they receive it?

PPSV23 is recommended for children with an immunocompromising condition or functional or anatomic asplenia, and also for immunocompetent children with chronic heart disease, chronic lung disease, diabetes mellitus, cerebrospinal fluid leak, or cochlear implant. Administer 1 dose of PPSV23 to children age 2 years and older at least 8 weeks after the child has received the final dose of PCV13. Children with an immunocompromising condition or functional or anatomic asplenia should receive a second dose of PPSV23 5 years after the first PPSV23.

Can you please explain when and why the recommendations for vaccination were changed for people with asthma and for cigarette smokers?

In 2008, the Advisory Committee on Immunization Practices (ACIP) reviewed information suggesting that asthma is an independent risk factor for pneumococcal disease among adults. ACIP also reviewed information that demonstrated an increased risk of pneumococcal disease among smokers. Consequently, ACIP recommended the inclusion of both asthma and cigarette smoking as risk factors for pneumococcal disease among adults age 19 through 64 years and as indications for PPSV23. However, pneumococcal conjugate vaccine (PCV13) is *not* recommended for persons whose only risk factor for invasive pneumococcal disease is asthma or cigarette smoking.

Is pneumococcal polysaccharide vaccine (PPSV23, Pneumovax; Merck) indicated for former smokers?

PPSV23 is currently recommended for people age 19 through 64 years who actively smoke cigarettes (see www.cdc.gov/mmwr/preview/mmwrhtml/mm5934a3.htm). However, chronic lung disease is an indication for PPSV23, and this could be applicable for former smokers.

Pneumococcal polysaccharide vaccine is recommended for people with diabetes. Does this include gestational diabetes?

No.

Which adults age 19–64 years should receive a second dose of PPSV23?

A second PPSV23 given 5 years after the first dose is recommended for people age 19 through 64 years who have functional or anatomic asplenia (including persons with sickle cell disease or splenectomy patients) or chronic renal failure (including dialysis patients) or nephrotic syndrome; are immunocompromised, including those with HIV infection, leukemia, lymphoma, Hodgkin's disease, multiple myeloma, or generalized malignancy; are receiving immunosuppressive therapy (including long-term systemic corticosteroids or radiation therapy); or who have received a solid organ transplant.

During an office visit, can a health care provider administer PCV13 and PPSV23 to an adult patient who needs both vaccines but has had neither? If not, what is the recommended interval between doses?

PCV13 and PPSV23 should not be given at the same visit. Patients who need both PCV13 and PPSV23 and who have received neither should receive PCV13 first, followed by a dose of PPSV23 at least 8 weeks later. If a second PPSV23 dose is recommended, it should be administered at least 5 years after the first PPSV23 dose.

Which adults are now recommended to receive a dose of PCV13?

In 2014, ACIP recommended routine vaccination with one dose of PCV13 for all persons at age 65 years who have not previously received PCV13 or whose PCV13 vaccination history is unknown. PPSV23 recommendations have not changed, so PCV13 and PPSV23 should both be administered at age 65 years. PCV13 should be administered 6 to 12 months before PPSV23 if possible. Persons who have already received PPSV23 should receive PCV13 12 months after PPSV23. PCV13 and PPSV23 should not be administered at the same visit.

In addition to adults age 65 years and older, adults age 19 through 64 years and older who have the conditions specified below and have not previously received PCV13 should receive a PCV13 dose during their next vaccination opportunity.

- Immunocompromising conditions (e.g., congenital or acquired immunodeficiency, HIV, chronic renal failure, nephrotic syndrome, leukemia, lymphoma, Hodgkin's disease, generalized malignancy, iatrogenic immunosuppression, solid organ transplant, multiple myeloma)
- Functional or anatomic asplenia (e.g., sickle cell disease and other hemoglobinopathies, congenital and acquired asplenia)
- Cerebrospinal fluid (CSF) leak
- Cochlear implants

Tetanus, Diphtheria, and Pertussis

At what gestational age of pregnancy should we vaccinate pregnant women with Tdap (tetanus toxoid, reduced diphtheria toxoid, and acellular pertussis vaccine, adsorbed)?

To maximize maternal antibody response and passive antibody transfer to the infant, the optimal time to administer Tdap is between 27 and 36 weeks' gestation. However, Tdap can be administered at any time during pregnancy. Previously, CDC had recommended that Tdap vaccination occur after 20 weeks' gestation.

Should further doses of pertussis vaccine be given to an infant or child who has had culture-proven pertussis?

Immunity to pertussis following infection is not lifelong. Persons with a history of pertussis should continue to receive pertussis-containing vaccines according to the recommended schedule. (Note: This answer is based on recommendations of the American Academy of Pediatrics Committee on Infectious Diseases.)

When should a person receive tetanus toxoid (TT) alone?
Single-antigen tetanus toxoid should be used only in rare instances, such as when a person has had a documented severe allergic response to diphtheria toxoid.

Is there an upper age limit for Tdap administration? For example, should I vaccinate an 85-year-old?
There is no upper age limit for Tdap vaccination. A single dose of Tdap is recommended for all adults.

If a health care worker receives Tdap vaccine and is then exposed to someone with pertussis, do you treat the vaccinated worker with prophylactic antibiotics or consider the worker immune to pertussis?
You should follow the postexposure prophylaxis protocol for pertussis exposure recommended by CDC (www.cdc.gov/vaccines/pubs/pertussis-guide/guide.htm). Research is needed to evaluate the effectiveness of Tdap for preventing pertussis in health care settings. Until studies define the optimal management of exposed vaccinated health care personnel, or experts arrive at consensus, health care facilities should continue to follow the postexposure prophylaxis protocol for vaccinated workers who are exposed to pertussis.

Someone gave Tdap to an infant instead of DTaP (diphtheria and tetanus toxoids and acellular pertussis vaccine, adsorbed). Now what should be done?
If Tdap is inadvertently administered to a child, it should not be counted as the first, second, or third dose of DTaP. You should repeat the dose with DTaP and continue vaccinating on schedule. If the dose of Tdap was administered for the fourth or fifth DTaP dose, the Tdap dose can be counted as valid. Please remind your staff to always check and double check the vaccine vial before administering any vaccine.

Varicella and Zoster

In patients age 60 or older who don't remember having chickenpox in the past, should we test for varicella immunity before giving zoster vaccine?

No. Vaccinate them with zoster vaccine according to the ACIP recommendations without serologic testing.

Can you catch shingles from a person with active shingles infection?

Shingles cannot be passed from one person to another through sneezing, coughing, or casual contact. If a person who has never had chickenpox or been vaccinated against chickenpox comes in direct contact with a shingles rash, the virus could be transmitted to the susceptible person. The exposed person would develop chickenpox, not shingles.

Should a person who has received two doses of varicella vaccine be vaccinated with zoster vaccine at age 60?

No. CDC does not currently recommend zoster vaccine for people who have received two doses of varicella vaccine. However, health care providers do not need to inquire about varicella vaccination history before administering zoster vaccine, because virtually all people currently or soon to be in the recommended age group have not received varicella vaccine. For details, see the CDC recommendations for prevention of herpes zoster, available at www.cdc.gov/mmwr/PDF/rr/rr5705.pdf.

If a person develops a rash after receiving varicella vaccination, does the vaccinee need to be isolated from susceptible people who are either pregnant or immunosuppressed?

Transmission of varicella vaccine virus is rare. However, if a pregnant or immunosuppressed household contact of a vaccinated person is known to be susceptible to varicella, and if the vaccinee develops a rash 7 to 21 days following vaccination, it is prudent for the vaccinee to avoid prolonged close contact with the susceptible person until the rash resolves.

Zoster vaccine is approved by FDA for people age 50 years and older. Does ACIP recommend that clinicians vaccinate people in their 50s?

At its October 2013 meeting, ACIP reviewed the current status of zoster vaccine licensure and the burden of herpes zoster (HZ) disease. ACIP declined to vote to expand the recommendations for the use of zoster vaccine to include people age 50 through 59 years for the following reasons: (1) though the burden of HZ disease increases after age 50, disease rates are lower in this age group than they are in persons age 60 years and older; (2) there is insufficient evidence for long-term protection provided by the vaccine; and (3) persons vaccinated at an age younger than 60 may not be protected when the incidence of zoster and its complications is highest. However, since zoster vaccine is approved by FDA for persons age 50 through 59 years, clinicians may vaccinate persons in this age group without an ACIP recommendation.

How soon after a case of shingles can a person receive zoster vaccine?
The general guideline for any vaccine is to wait until the acute stage of the illness is over and symptoms abate. However, a recent case of shingles is expected to boost the person's immunity to varicella. Zoster vaccine is also intended to boost immunity to varicella. Administering zoster vaccine to a person whose immunity was recently boosted by a case of shingles might reduce the effectiveness of the vaccine. ACIP does not have a specific recommendation on this issue, but it may be prudent to defer zoster vaccination for 6 to 12 months after the shingles has resolved so that the vaccine can produce a more effective boost to immunity.

The Zostavax package insert says to inject the vaccine into the deltoid region of the upper arm. We always give subcutaneous vaccines in the triceps area of the arm. Is this wrong?
No. The subcutaneous tissue overlying the triceps muscle of the upper arm is the usual location for subcutaneous vaccine injection for an adult.

When can a patient previously on immunosuppressive chemotherapy receive zoster vaccine?
If the patient was on anticancer therapy, wait 3 months. If the person was on high-dose corticosteroids, isoantibodies, immune-system mediators, or immunomodulators, wait 1 month. If the person was on low doses of methotrexate, azathioprine, or mercaptopurine, waiting is not indicated because these are not considered immunosuppressive. See the ACIP recommendations for zoster at www.cdc.gov/mmwr/pdf/rr/rr5705.pdf for details.

Pregnancy and Breast-feeding

Can thimerosal-containing vaccine be given to pregnant women?
Yes, unless you live in a state that has enacted legislation restricting use in pregnant women. There is no scientific evidence that thimerosal in vaccines, including influenza vaccines, is a cause of adverse events, unless the patient has a systemic allergy to thimerosal.

For how long should a woman of childbearing age avoid pregnancy after receiving a live attenuated vaccine?
Because of theoretical risks to the developing fetus, ACIP recommends that women avoid pregnancy for 4 weeks after receiving a live attenuated vaccine (e.g., MMR, varicella, LAIV). This interval may be shorter than that recommended by the manufacturer.

Is there a risk for a pregnant staff person administering live virus vaccines?
A pregnant woman may administer any vaccine except smallpox vaccine.

Is it acceptable to give breast-feeding mothers Tdap vaccine?
Yes. Women who have never received Tdap and who did not receive it during pregnancy should receive it immediately postpartum or as soon as possible thereafter.

Which vaccines can be given to breast-feeding women?
All vaccines except smallpox can be given to breast-feeding women. Breast-feeding is a precaution for yellow fever vaccine. Women who are breast-feeding should be advised to postpone travel to yellow fever endemic or epidemic regions; however, if travel cannot be postponed, the woman should receive yellow fever vaccine.

Thimerosal and Aluminum

Does the thimerosal in some of the injectable influenza vaccines pose a risk?
Thimerosal, a very effective preservative, has been used to prevent bacterial contamination in vaccine vials for more than 50 years. It contains a type of mercury known as ethylmercury, which is different from the type of mercury found in fish and seafood (methylmercury). At very high

levels, methylmercury can be toxic to people, especially to the neurologic development of infants.

In recent years, several large scientific studies have determined that thimerosal in vaccines does not lead to neurologic problems, such as autism. Nonetheless, because we generally try to reduce people's exposure to mercury if at all possible, vaccine manufacturers have voluntarily changed their production methods to produce vaccines that are now free of thimerosal or have only trace amounts. They have done this because it is possible to do, not because there was any evidence that the thimerosal was harmful.

Is there any evidence that MMR or thimerosal causes autism?
No. This issue has been studied extensively in recent years, including a thorough review by the independent Institute of Medicine (IOM). The IOM issued a report in 2004 that concluded there is no evidence supporting an association between MMR vaccine or thimerosal-containing vaccines and the development of autism. To access the IOM committee minutes, as well as the executive summaries and full reports, go to www.iom.edu/Reports/2004/immunization-safety-review-vaccines-and-autism.aspx. To obtain more information on thimerosal and vaccines in general, visit www.cdc.org/vaccinesafety/concerns/thimerosal/index.html.

Many of my patients are reading* The Vaccine Book, *in which the author, Dr. Robert W. Sears, cites studies that he interprets as showing that the amount of aluminum found in certain vaccines might be unsafe. He thinks it is better to separate aluminum-containing vaccines, rather than give them according to the recommended U.S. immunization schedule. I would love any information you have about this.
Paul Offit, MD, and Charlotte Moser, BS, of the Vaccine Education Center (VEC) at the Children's Hospital of Philadelphia, published an article, "The Problem with Dr. Bob's Alternative Vaccine Schedule," in the January 2009 issue of *Pediatrics.* It includes a section about aluminum. You can read the article in its entirety at http://pediatrics.aappublications.org/cgi/content/full/123/1/e164.

Here are some additional sources of related information:

- "Aluminum in Vaccines: What you should know" is available from VEC at www.chop.edu/export/download/pdfs/articles/vaccine-education-center/aluminum.pdf.
- "Vaccine Ingredients: What you should know" is available from VEC at www.chop.edu/export/download/pdfs/articles/vaccine-education-center/vaccine-ingredients.pdf.
- "Questions and Answers about Vaccine Ingredients" is available from the American Academy of Pediatrics at www.aap.org/immunization/families/faq/Vaccineingredients.pdf.

Latex Allergy and Anaphylaxis

What precautions should we take for patients who have a latex allergy?

Severe anaphylactic reactions to latex are rare, but people who have had such a reaction should generally not be given vaccines that have been in contact with natural rubber unless the benefit of vaccination outweighs the risk of a potential allergic reaction. People with latex allergies that are not anaphylactic may be vaccinated as usual; included in this category are contact-type allergies, such as a reaction that occurs with prolonged contact with latex-containing gloves.

If we have a patient with a severe latex allergy, why shouldn't we just remove the stopper from the vial before withdrawing the vaccine in order to prevent a latex reaction?

The patient should not be given the vaccine from that vial. We do not recommend removing the stopper from a vaccine vial and administering the vaccine to a person who has a severe, life-threatening allergy to latex. The vaccine has already been exposed to the rubber stopper in the vial, which might be just enough exposure to cause a reaction.

What percentage of vaccine recipients will experience an anaphylactic reaction?

It is estimated that for every 1 million doses administered, about 1 dose (~0.0001%) will result in an anaphylactic reaction after vaccination. With proper screening, most providers who administer thousands of vaccines in their lifetimes will never see an anaphylactic reaction.

Vaccine Administration

What should we do if we give an injection by the wrong route, for example, intramuscularly (IM) instead of subcutaneously (SC)?

Vaccines should always be given by the route recommended by the manufacturer, because data on the safety and efficacy of alternative routes are limited. If this does inadvertently happen, ACIP recommends that vaccines given by the wrong route be counted as valid with three exceptions: hepatitis B, rabies, or HPV vaccine given by any route other than IM should not be counted as valid and should be repeated. This and other information on vaccine administration is discussed in the ACIP "General Recommendations on Immunization" (www.cdc.gov/vaccines/pubs/acip-list.htm).

What does "simultaneous administration of vaccines" mean? Does it mean the same day, the same hour, or what?

Simultaneous means the same day—the same clinic day. If someone receives a vaccine in the morning and then another that same afternoon, it would be considered simultaneous administration.

Why are some vaccinations given subcutaneously (SC) while others must be given intramuscularly (IM)?

In general, vaccines containing adjuvants (components that enhance the antigenic response) are administered IM to avoid irritation, induration, skin discoloration, inflammation, and granuloma formation if injected into subcutaneous tissue. This includes most of the inactivated vaccines, with a few exceptions (such as IPV and pneumococcal vaccines, which may be given either SC or IM). In addition, a vaccine's efficacy may be reduced if it is not given by the recommended route.

A 5-year-old came in today for her preschool vaccines. She needed MMR and varicella. She has a broken arm, which is in a cast. Can the anterolateral thigh be used to administer a subcutaneous vaccine to a 5-year-old?

Yes. There is no age limit for use of the anterolateral thigh for either subcutaneous or intramuscular vaccines.

Some single-dose manufacturer-filled vaccines come with an air pocket in the syringe chamber. Do we need to expel the air pocket before vaccinating?

No. You do not need to expel the air pocket. The air will be absorbed. This is not true for syringes that you fill yourself; you should expel air bubbles from these syringes before vaccination to the extent that you can do so.

The cap of a single-dose vial (SDV) of vaccine was removed and the stopper cleaned, but before the needle was inserted it was discovered to be the incorrect vaccine. Can a SDV be stored and used at a later time if no needle has been inserted into the vial stopper even though the cap has been removed?

The current CDC recommendation is that when a single-dose vial or syringe has been "activated," meaning the protective cap has been removed, the dose must be used during that clinic session or else it should be discarded, even if the vial has not been punctured with a needle.

In cleaning the vaccine vial stopper or the patient's skin, is it okay to use a nonsterile cotton ball or do we need to use a prepackaged sterile alcohol prep pad?

Using a prepackaged sterile alcohol prep pad is recommended to maintain aseptic technique. Not only are cotton balls not sterile; neither is a bottle of sterile alcohol, once it's opened.

Some single-dose vials (SDV) contain more than the recommended dosage of the vaccine. For example, drawing up the entire SDV of HPV4 yields about 0.6 mL of vaccine. Should we administer the recommended dose of the vaccine, or administer the entire contents of the vial even if the volume exceeds the recommended dose?

The entire volume should be used even if it is a little more than 0.5 mL. Discarding the excess vaccine is not required or recommended.

If I have to give more than one injection in a muscle, are certain vaccines best given together?

Since DTaP and pneumococcal conjugate are the vaccines most likely to cause a local reaction, it is practical to give DTaP and PCV in separate limbs (if possible) so there is no confusion about which vaccine caused the reaction.

What are the special recommendations for administering intramuscular injections in people with clotting disorders?

This issue is discussed in the ACIP "General Recommendations on Immunization" (www.cdc.gov/vaccines/pubs/acip-list.htm). IM injections should be scheduled shortly after antihemophilia therapy or just before a dose of anticoagulant. For both IM and subcutaneous injections, a fine needle (23 gauge or smaller) should be used and firm pressure should be applied to the site, without rubbing, for at least 2 minutes. Providers should not administer a vaccine by a route that is not approved by FDA for that particular vaccine (e.g., administration of IM vaccines by the subcutaneous route).

Is changing needles after a vaccine dose has been drawn into a syringe recommended?

No. Also, it is unnecessary to change the needle if it has passed through two stoppers, which occurs when a lyophilized vaccine is reconstituted. Changing needles is a waste of resources and increases the risk of needlestick injury.

Do you need to aspirate before giving a vaccination?

No. ACIP does not recommend aspiration when administering vaccines, because no data exist to justify the need for this practice. IM injections are not given in areas where large vessels are present. Given the size of the needle and the angle at which you inject the vaccine, it is difficult to cannulate a vessel without rupturing it and even more difficult to actually deliver the vaccine intravenously. We are aware of no reports of a vaccine being administered intravenously and causing harm in the absence of aspiration.

If some portion of a vaccine (e.g., influenza vaccine) leaks out of the syringe while it is injected into a patient, does the dose need to be repeated and, if so, when?

When this happens, it is difficult to judge how much vaccine the person received. This would be a nonstandard dose and should not be counted. You should go ahead and re-immunize the individual at that time.

Is it safe to give a vaccine directly into an area where there is a tattoo?

Both IM and subcutaneous vaccines may be given through a tattoo.

If two live virus vaccines are inadvertently given less than 4 weeks apart, what should be done?

If two live virus vaccines are administered less than 4 weeks apart and not on the same day, the vaccine given second should be considered invalid and repeated. The repeat dose should be administered at least 4 weeks after the invalid dose. Alternatively, one can perform serologic testing to check for immunity, but this option may be more costly.

Vaccine Storage and Expiration Dates

For an extended period, the temperature in the vaccine-storage refrigerator in our practice was too cold. We assume all the vaccines given during that period are considered invalid. How should we schedule the revaccinations?

If administered vaccine is found to have been stored at an inappropriate temperature, the provider should contact the state health department to determine whether the vaccine dose is invalid. If the vaccine dose is determined to be invalid, another dose should be given. This applies to inactivated or live vaccines. If the damaged vaccine was a live virus vaccine (e.g., MMR, varicella), you should wait at least 4 weeks after the previous (damaged) dose was given before repeating it. If the damaged vaccine was an inactivated vaccine, you can give the repeat dose on the same day you gave the damaged dose or at any other time. If you prefer, you can perform serologic testing to check for immunity for certain vaccinations (e.g., measles, rubella, hepatitis A, tetanus).

I've heard that multidose vaccine vials should be disposed of after being open for 30 days. Is this true?

No. Multidose vials of vaccine that do not require reconstitution may be used through the expiration date printed on the label or box as long as the vaccine is not visibly contaminated, unless otherwise specified by the manufacturer.

When the expiration date of a vaccine indicates a month and year, does the vaccine expire on the first or last day of the month?

Vaccine may be used through the last day of the month indicated in the expiration date. After that, do not use it. Monitor your vaccine supply carefully so that vaccines do not expire.

We have a small office with limited space for a vaccine storage unit. If dormitory-style refrigerators are no longer an option, what can we use?

A dormitory-style refrigerator is a small combination refrigerator/ freezer unit that is outfitted with one exterior door and an evaporator plate (cooling coil), which is usually located inside an icemaker compartment (freezer) within the refrigerator. This type of unit has severe temperature control and stability issues. However, compact "purpose built" or "pharmacy grade" refrigerators and freezers that have been engineered to maintain even temperatures throughout the unit are available, and these are ideal for use in small offices. In general, the unit must be large enough to store the year's largest vaccine inventory without crowding and to store water bottles (in a refrigerator) and frozen coolant packs (in a freezer) to stabilize the temperatures and minimize fluctuations.

Since I am no longer storing frozen vaccines in the freezer portion of my combination refrigerator/freezer, should I just turn off the freezer portion of the unit?

No. If you turn off the freezer portion of a combination refrigerator/ freezer, the refrigerated compartment will not maintain the proper temperature.

Is it okay to store medications and other biologic products in the same unit as vaccines?

According to CDC's Vaccine Storage and Handling Toolkit, other medications and biologic products should be stored in separate units from vaccines. If the same unit must be used, these products should be stored below the vaccines on a different shelf. This will reduce the risk of medication errors and prevent contamination of the vaccines should the other products spill.

Miscellaneous

What is meant by "minimum intervals" between vaccine doses?

Vaccination schedules are generally determined by clinical trials, usually prior to licensure of the vaccine. The spacing of doses in the clinical trial usually becomes the recommended schedule. A "minimum interval" is shorter than the recommended interval; it is the shortest time between two doses of a vaccine series in which an adequate response to the second dose can be expected. The concern is that a dose given too soon after the previous dose may reduce the response. The minimum spacing between doses is generally included in the ACIP statement for that vaccine. In addition, an extensive list of recommended and minimum intervals and ages for vaccination can be found in Table 1 of ACIP's "General Recommendations on Immunization" (www.cdc.gov/vaccines/pubs/ACIP-list.htm).

Are vaccine diluents interchangeable?

As a general rule, vaccine diluents are not interchangeable. One exception is that the diluent for MMR can be used to reconstitute varicella vaccine, and vice versa. The diluent for both vaccines, produced by the same company, is sterile water for injection. No other diluent can be used for MMR and varicella vaccines, and these diluents must not be used to reconstitute any other lyophilized vaccine.

We frequently see patients who are febrile or have an acute illness and are due for vaccinations. We're never quite sure whether we should withhold the vaccines. What do you advise?

A "moderate or severe acute illness" is a precaution for administering any vaccine. A mild acute illness (e.g., diarrhea, mild upper-respiratory tract infection) with or without fever is not. The concern in vaccinating someone with moderate or severe illness is that a fever following the vaccine could complicate management of the concurrent illness (that is, it could be difficult to determine if the fever was from the vaccine or due to the concurrent illness). In deciding whether to vaccinate a patient with moderate or severe illness, the clinician needs to determine whether forgoing vaccination will increase the patient's risk for vaccine-preventable diseases, as is the case if the patient is unlikely to return for vaccination or to seek vaccination elsewhere.

Some parents are requesting that we space out their infants' vaccinations because they are concerned that receiving multiple vaccinations at a single office visit might overwhelm the infant's immune system. What do you think about using alternative schedules?

Vaccine recommendations are determined after extensive studies in large clinical trials. They include studies on how vaccine recipients respond to multiple vaccines given simultaneously. The overall aim is to provide early protection for infants and children against vaccine-preventable diseases that could endanger their health and life. There is no scientific evidence supporting a benefit from delaying vaccinations or separating them into individual antigens. Rather, this practice prolongs susceptibility to disease and could result in a greater likelihood of the child becoming sick with a serious or life-threatening illness. There could also be added expense (e.g., multiple office visits), additional time off from work for parents, and increased likelihood that the child will fail to get all necessary vaccinations.

Where can I find names of vaccines used outside the United States?

Appendix B of the CDC publication *Epidemiology and Prevention of Vaccine-Preventable Diseases* (The Pink Book) lists names for vaccines used outside the United States. You'll find Appendix B at www.cdc.gov/vaccines/pubs/pinkbook/downloads/appendices/B/foreign-products-tables.pdf.

Why aren't people in the United States vaccinated with BCG?

BCG vaccine is used in countries of high endemicity to help prevent tuberculosis disease. A more effective strategy for the prevention of tuberculosis in countries where the endemicity is low is to identify infected persons by using a Mantoux (PPD) skin test and to eliminate the infection with antituberculous drugs. This is the strategy used in the United States.

Why do ACIP recommendations not always agree with package inserts?

There is usually very close agreement between vaccine package inserts and ACIP statements. FDA must approve the package insert, and the agency requires documentation for all claims and recommendations made in the insert. Occasionally, ACIP may use different data to formulate its recommendations or may try to add flexibility to its recommendations, which results in wording different from that on the package insert. ACIP sometimes makes recommendations on the basis of expert opinion and public health considerations. Published recommendations of national advisory groups (such as ACIP or the American Academy of Pediatrics Committee on Infectious Diseases) should be considered equally as authoritative as those on the package insert.

If my state has an immunization information system (IIS, or registry) do I still need to give the patient a vaccine record card?

Yes. Patient-held cards are an extremely important part of a person's medical history. The person may move to an area without a registry, and the personal record may be the only vaccination record available. In addition, even within a state, all health care providers may not participate in the registry, so the personal record card would be needed.

Chapter 19

Vaccine Product Information

The vaccine product information presented here is based on the routine recommended dosing schedules for commonly used vaccines. Alternative dosing schedules may be available for select vaccines. Also, dosing concentrations may vary for vaccines available from different manufacturers. Consult the package inserts for detailed dosing information. Current procedural terminology (CPT®) codes have been provided for the most common routes and schedules; other codes may exist for specific circumstances. CPT® codes are copyright © 2013, American Medical Association, printed here under "fair use" provisions.

Not all vaccines licensed for distribution in the United States have been included. Consult the manufacturers' prescribing information and CDC resources for information on vaccines not included in this section.

Remember to always check expiration dates before administering vaccines. These vary not only by lot number but also by vaccine type. Follow manufacturer guidance for the shelf life of reconstituted vaccine and multidose vaccine vials.

Information is presented here on the following vaccines:

Diphtheria & Tetanus Toxoids Adsorbed (DT)

Vaccine type: Inactivated
Age indications: Children 6 weeks to 7 years
Preparation: Shake well
Storage: Store at 2°C–8°C (35°F–46°F); do not freeze
Shelf life once reconstituted: N/A
Volume and route: 0.5 mL IM
Dosing schedule: Refer to the product package inserts and immunization schedules provided by CDC
Contraindications: Severe allergic reaction to a previous dose or vaccine component
Precautions: Occurrence of Guillain-Barré syndrome in <6 weeks following a previous dose of tetanus-containing vaccine; moderate or severe acute illness with or without fever; history of Arthus-type hypersensitivity reaction following previous dose of tetanus or diphtheria-toxoid containing vaccine (including MCV4)—defer vaccination for at least 10 years
CPT code: 90702

Trade name: None
Manufacturer: Sanofi Pasteur
Product specifications: Single-dose vial (10 per package); rubber stopper contains latex
NDC: 49281-0278-10

Additional dose interchangeability: N/A

References

Centers for Disease Control and Prevention. Errata: Vol. 60, No. RR-2. *MMWR Morb Mortal Wkly Rep.* 2011;60:993.

Centers for Disease Control and Prevention. General recommendations on immunization: recommendations of the Advisory Committee on Immunization Practices (ACIP). *MMWR Recomm Rep.* 2011: 60(RR-2);1–60.

Diphtheria and Tetanus Toxoids Adsorbed USP [package insert]. Swiftwater, PA: Sanofi Pasteur; December 2005.

Immunization Action Coalition. Guide to contraindications and precautions to commonly used vaccines. www.immunize.org/catg.d/p3072a.pdf. Accessed October 13, 2014.

Diphtheria & Tetanus Toxoids & Acellular Pertussis Vaccine Adsorbed (DTaP)

Vaccine type: Inactivated
Age indications: 6 weeks to 7 years
Preparation: Shake well
Storage: Store at 2°C–8°C (35°F–46°F); do not freeze
Shelf life once reconstituted: N/A
Volume and route: 0.5 mL IM
Dosing schedule: Refer to the product package inserts and immunization schedules provided by CDC
Contraindications: Severe allergic reaction to previous dose or vaccine component; encephalopathy not attributable to another identifiable cause within 7 days following administration of previous dose of DTP [diphtheria and tetanus toxoids and whole-cell pertussis vaccine] or DTaP
Precautions: Temperature ≥40.5°C (≥105°F), collapse or shock-like state, or persistent, inconsolable crying lasting ≥3 hours within 48 hours following a previous dose; seizure within 3 days following previous dose; Guillain-Barré syndrome <6 weeks following previous dose of tetanus-containing vaccine; moderate or severe acute illness with or without fever; history of Arthus-type hypersensitivity reaction following previous dose of tetanus or diphtheria-toxoid containing vaccine (including MCV4)—defer vaccination for at least 10 years; progressive or unstable neurologic disorder (defer DTaP until condition stabilizes); latex allergy—Infanrix prefilled syringe
CPT code: 90700

Trade name: Daptacel
Manufacturer: Sanofi Pasteur
Product specifications: Single-dose vial
NDC: 49281-0286-01 (1 per package); 49281-0286-05 (5 per package); 49281-0286-10 (10 per package)

Trade name: Infanrix
Manufacturer: GlaxoSmithKline
Product specifications: Single-dose vial
NDC: 58160-0810-01 (1 per package); 58160-0810-11 (10 per package)
Product specifications: Prefilled syringe (no latex in plunger; tip cap may contain latex)
NDC: 58160-0810-43 (1 per package); 58160-0810-52 (10 per package)

Additional dose interchangeability: Not recommended, because of lack of study data

References

Centers for Disease Control and Prevention. Errata: Vol. 60, No. RR-2. *MMWR Morb Mortal Wkly Rep.* 2011;60:993.

Centers for Disease Control and Prevention. General recommendations on immunization: recommendations of the Advisory Committee on Immunization Practices (ACIP). *MMWR Recomm Rep.* 2011: 60(RR-2);1–60.

Daptacel [package insert]. Swiftwater, PA: Sanofi Pasteur; October 2013.

Immunization Action Coalition. Guide to contraindications and precautions to commonly used vaccines. www.immunize.org/catg.d/p3072a.pdf. Accessed October 13, 2014.

Infanrix [package insert]. Research Triangle Park, NC: GlaxoSmithKline; November 2013.

Haemophilus b Conjugate Vaccine

Vaccine type: Inactivated
Age indications: ActHIB—2 to 18 months
PedvaxHIB—2 to 71 months
Hiberix—15 months through 4 years
Preparation: ActHIB—Reconstitute
PedvaxHIB—Shake well
Hiberix—Reconstitute
Storage: Store at 2°C–8°C (35°F–46°F); do not freeze
Shelf life once reconstituted: ActHIB and Hiberix—24 hours
Volume and route: 0.5 mL IM
Dosing schedule: ActHIB and PedvaxHIB—Refer to the product package inserts and immunization schedules provided by CDC
Hiberix—to be used as a booster dose
Contraindications: Severe allergic reaction to previous dose or vaccine component; age less than 6 weeks
Precautions: Moderate or severe acute illness with or without fever; latex allergy—ActHIB diluent vial, Hiberix prefilled syringe, PedvaxHIB vial
ActHIB and Hiberix—Guillian-Barré syndrome <6 weeks following previous dose of tetanus-containing vaccine
CPT code: ActHIB and Hiberix—90648
PedvaxHIB—90647

Trade name: ActHIB
Manufacturer: Sanofi Pasteur
Product specifications: Single-dose lyophilized vaccine plus diluent (5 per package); diluent vial stopper contains latex
NDC: 42981-0545-05

Trade name: Liquid PedvaxHIB
Manufacturer: Merck
Product specifications: Single-dose vial (10 per package); vial stopper contains latex
NDC: 00006-4897-00

Trade name: Hiberix
Manufacturer: GlaxoSmithKline
Product specifications: Single-dose vial of lyophilized vaccine
NDC: 58160-0806-01 (1 per package); 58160-0806-05 (10 per package)
Product specifications: Prefilled syringe with diluents; tip cap may contain latex
NDC: 58160-0951-02 (1 per package); 58160-0951-11 (10 per package)

Additional dose interchangeability: ActiHIB and PedvaxHIB can be interchanged; Hiberix is used as a booster dose, not primary immunization

References

ActHIB [package insert]. Swiftwater, PA: Sanofi Pasteur; January 2014.

Centers for Disease Control and Prevention. General recommendations on immunization: recommendations of the Advisory Committee on Immunization Practices (ACIP). *MMWR Recomm Rep.* 2011: 60(RR-2);1–60.

Hiberix [package insert]. Research Triangle Park, NC: GlaxoSmithKline; March 2012.

Immunization Action Coalition. Guide to contraindications and precautions to commonly used vaccines. www.immunize.org/catg.d/p3072a.pdf. Accessed October 13, 2014.

Liquid PedvaxHIB [package insert]. West Point, PA: Merck; December 2010.

Hepatitis A Vaccine

Vaccine type: Inactivated
Age indications: 12 months through adult
Preparation: Shake well
Storage: Store at 2°C–8°C (35°F–46°F); do not freeze
Shelf life once reconstituted: N/A
Volume and route: ≥12 months through 18 years—0.5 mL IM
Adults >18 years—1 mL IM
Dosing schedule: Two doses, 6 to 12 months apart (HAVRIX) or 6 to 18 months apart (VAQTA)
Contraindications: Severe allergic reaction to previous dose or vaccine component; HAVRIX and VAQTA contain neomycin
Precautions: Moderate or severe acute illness with or without fever; latex allergy—HAVRIX prefilled syringe, VAQTA prefilled syringe and vial
CPT code: Two-dose pediatric—90633
Adult—90632

Trade name: HAVRIX
Manufacturer: GlaxoSmithKline
Product specifications: 0.5 mL single-dose vial
NDC: 58160-0825-01 (1 per package); 58160-0825-11 (10 per package)
Product specifications: 0.5 mL prefilled syringe (tip cap may contain latex)
NDC: 58160-0825-43 (1 per package); 58160-0825-52 (10 per package)
Product specifications: 1 mL single-dose vial
NDC: 58160-0826-01 (1 per package); 58160-0826-11 (10 per package)
Product specifications: 1 mL prefilled syringe (tip cap may contain latex)
NDC: 58160-0826-34 (1 per package); 58160-0826-52 (10 per package)

Trade name: VAQTA
Manufacturer: Merck
Product specifications: 0.5 mL single-dose vial; vial stopper contains latex
NDC: 00006-4831-41 (10 per package)
Product specifications: 0.5 mL prefilled syringe; tip cap and plunger contain latex
NDC: 00006-4095-09 (6 per package); 00006-4095-02 (10 per package)
Product specifications: 1 mL single-dose vial; vial stopper contains latex
NDC: 00006-4841-00 (1 per package); 00006-4841-41 (10 per package)
Product specifications: 1 mL prefilled syringe; tip cap and plunger contain latex
NDC: 00006-4096-09 (6 per package); 00006-4096-02 (10 per package)

Additional dose interchangeability: Products can be interchanged

References

Centers for Disease Control and Prevention. General recommendations on immunization: recommendations of the Advisory Committee on Immunization Practices (ACIP). *MMWR Recomm Rep.* 2011: 60(RR-2);1–60.

HAVRIX [package insert]. Research Triangle Park, NC: GlaxoSmithKline; July 2014.

Immunization Action Coalition. Guide to contraindications and precautions to commonly used vaccines. www.immunize.org/catg.d/p3072a.pdf. Accessed October 13, 2014.

VAQTA [package insert]. West Point, PA: Merck; February 2014.

Hepatitis B Vaccine

Vaccine type: Inactivated
Age indications: Birth through adulthood
Preparation: Shake well
Storage: Store at 2°C–8°C (35°F–46°F); do not freeze
Shelf life once reconstituted: N/A
Volume and route: Birth through 19 years—0.5 mL IM
>19 years—1 mL IM
Dosing schedule: Three doses at month 0, month 1, month 6
Contraindications: Severe allergic reaction to previous dose or vaccine component; Engerix-B and Recombivax HB contain yeast
Precautions: Moderate or severe acute illness with or without fever; infants weighing <2000 grams; latex allergy—Engerix-B prefilled syringe, Recombivax HB vial and prefilled syringe
CPT code: Three-dose pediatric—90744
Two-dose adolescent—90743
Three-dose adult—90746

Trade name: Engerix-B
Manufacturer: GlaxoSmithKline
Product specifications: 0.5 mL single-dose vial
NDC: 58160-0820-01 (1 per package); 58160-0820-11 (10 per package)
Product specifications: 0.5 mL prefilled syringe (tip cap may contain latex)
NDC: 58160-0820-43 (1 per package); 58160-0820-52 (10 per package)
Product specifications: 1 mL single-dose vial
NDC: 58160-0821-01 (1 per package); 58160-0821-11 (10 per package)
Product specifications: 1 mL prefilled syringe (tip cap may contain latex)
NDC: 58160-0821-34 (1 per package); 58160-0821-52 (10 per package)

Trade name: Recombivax HB*
Manufacturer: Merck
Product specifications: 0.5 mL single-dose vial; vial stopper contains latex
NDC: 00006-4981-00 (10 per package)
Product specifications: 0.5 mL prefilled syringe; tip cap and plunger contain latex
NDC: 00006-4093-09 (6 per package); 00006-4093-02 (10 per package)
Product specifications: 1 mL single-dose vial; vial stopper contains latex
NDC: 00006-4995-00 (1 per package); 00006-4995-41 (10 per package)
Product specifications: 1 mL prefilled syringe; tip cap and plunger contain latex
NDC: 00006-4094-09 (6 per package); 00006-4094-02 (10 per package)

*Contact the manufacturer for Dialysis Formulation information

Additional dose interchangeability: Products can be interchanged for three-dose schedule; Engerix-B is not FDA approved for two-dose schedule

References

Centers for Disease Control and Prevention. General recommendations on immunization: recommendations of the Advisory Committee on Immunization Practices (ACIP). *MMWR Recomm Rep.* 2011: 60(RR-2);1–60.

Engerix-B [package insert]. Research Triangle Park, NC: GlaxoSmithKline; December 2013.

Immunization Action Coalition. Guide to contraindications and precautions to commonly used vaccines. www.immunize.org/catg.d/p3072a.pdf. Accessed October 13, 2014.

Recombivax HB [package insert]. West Point, PA: Merck; May 2014.

Herpes Zoster Vaccine

Vaccine type: Live attenuated
Age indications: ≥50 years per FDA-approved indications; ≥60 years per ACIP recommendations
Preparation: Reconstitute (slowly inject diluent and gently agitate to avoid foaming)
Storage:[a] Store at –50°C to –15°C (–58°F to +5°F); do not freeze diluent; protect from light prior to reconstitution; do not ship using dry ice
Shelf life once reconstituted: 30 minutes
Volume and route: 0.65 mL subcutaneous
Dosing schedule: Single, one-time dose
Contraindications: Severe allergic reaction to previous dose or vaccine component (e.g., gelatin, neomycin); immunosuppression; pregnancy; active untreated tuberculosis
Precautions: Moderate or severe acute illness with or without fever; breast-feeding
Drug interactions: Antiviral medications used against herpes may reduce the effectiveness if given less than 24 hours prior to or within 14 days following vaccine. Although the manufacturer states concurrent administration of Zostavax and Pneumovax-23 can result in reduced immunogenicity of Zostavax, ACIP does not recommend waiting if both are needed
CPT code: 90736

[a]Zostavax products may be stored and/or transported at 2°–8°C (36°–46°F) for up to 72 continuous hours prior to reconstitution. If vaccine stored at this temperature is not used within 72 hours, it must be discarded.

Trade name: Zostavax
Manufacturer: Merck
Product specifications: Single-dose vial of lyophilized vaccine
NDC: 00006-4963-00 (1 per package plus 10 vials of diluent); 00006-4963-41 (10 per package plus 10 vials of diluent)

Additional dose interchangeability: N/A

References

Centers for Disease Control and Prevention. General recommendations on immunization: recommendations of the Advisory Committee on Immunization Practices (ACIP). *MMWR Recomm Rep.* 2011;60(RR-2):1–60.

Immunization Action Coalition. Guide to contraindications and precautions to commonly used vaccines. www.immunize.org/catg.d/p3072a.pdf. Accessed October 13, 2014.

Zostavax [package insert]. West Point, Pa: Merck; February 2014.

Human Papillomavirus Vaccine

Bivalent (Types 16 and 18), Quadrivalent (Types 6, 11, 16, and 18), 9-Valent (Types 6, 11, 16, 18, 31, 33, 45, 52, and 58)

Vaccine type: Inactivated

Age indications: Gardasil—9 through 26 years (females and males)
Gardasil 9—9 through 26 years (females) and 9 through 15 years (males)[a]
Cervarix—9 through 25 years (females)
Preparation: Shake well
Storage: Store at 2°C–8° C (35°F–46° F); do not freeze; protect from light
Shelf life once reconstituted: N/A
Volume and route: 0.5 mL IM
Dosing schedule: Three doses at month 0, month 1 or 2, month 6 (preferably at age 11 or 12 years)
Contraindications: Severe allergic reaction to previous dose or vaccine component (e.g., yeast—Gardasil)
Precautions: Moderate or severe acute illness with or without fever; pregnancy; latex allergy—Cervarix prefilled syringe
CPT code: Gardasil—90649
Gardasil 9—90651
Cervarix—90650

[a]As approved by FDA; ACIP recommendations pending.

Trade name: Bivalent—Cervarix
Manufacturer: GlaxoSmithKline
Product specifications: 0.5 mL prefilled syringe; tip cap contains latex
NDC: 58160-0830-05 (1 per package); 58160-0830-43 (10 per package)

Trade name: Quadrivalent—Gardasil
Manufacturer: Merck
Product specifications: 0.5 mL single-dose vial
NDC: 00006-4045-00 (1 per package); 00006-4045-41 (10 per package)
Product specifications: 0.5 mL prefilled syringe
NDC: 00006-4109-09 (6 per package); 00006-4109-02 (10 per package)

Trade name: 9-Valent—Gardasil 9
Manufacturer: Merck
Product specifications: 0.5 mL single-dose vial
NDC: 00006-4119-02 (1 per package); 00006-4119-03 (10 per package)
Product specifications: 0.5 mL prefilled syringe
NDC: 00006-4121-02 (10 per package)

Additional dose interchangeability: N/A

References

Centers for Disease Control and Prevention. General recommendations on immunization: recommendations of the Advisory Committee on Immunization Practices (ACIP). *MMWR Recomm Rep.* 2011;60(RR-2):1–60.

Centers for Disease Control and Prevention. Recommended adult immunization schedule—United States, 2014. www.cdc.gov/vaccines/schedules/hcp/adult.html. Accessed October 13, 2014.

Cervarix [package insert]. Research Triangle Park, NC: GlaxoSmithKline; July 2014.

Gardasil [package insert]. Whitehouse Station, NJ: Merck; June 2014.

Gardasil 9 [package insert]. Whitehouse Station, NJ: Merck; December 2014.

Immunization Action Coalition. Guide to contraindications and precautions to commonly used vaccines. www.immunize.org/catg.d/p3072a.pdf. Accessed October 13, 2014.

Merck. FDA approves Merck's HPV vaccine, Gardasil 9, to prevent cancers and other diseases caused by nine HPV types—including types that cause about 90% of cervical cancer cases. December 11, 2014. www.mercknewsroom.com/news-release/prescription-medicine-news/fda-approves-mercks-hpv-vaccine-gardasil9-prevent-cancers-an. Accessed December 22, 2014.

Inactivated Influenza Vaccine

Trivalent and Quadrivalent

Vaccine type: Inactivated
Age indications: Refer to table on pages 204–205
Preparation: Shake well; except FluBlok, which is a sterile solution
Storage: Store at 2°C–8°C (35°F–46°F); do not freeze; protect from light
Shelf life once reconstituted: N/A
Volume and route: 6 months through 35 months—0.25 mL IM; ≥36 months—0.5 mL IM
Fluzone Intradermal—0.1 mL (age 18–64 years)
Dosing schedule: 2 through 8 years—One or two doses,[a] 28 days apart; ≥9 years—annual
Contraindications: Severe allergic reaction to previous dose or vaccine component (e.g., egg;[b] neomycin—Afluria; polymixin B—Afluria)
Precautions: History of egg allergy resulting in hives only;[b] moderate or severe acute illness with or without fever; Guillain-Barré syndrome <6 weeks following previous dose of influenza vaccine; latex allergy—Flucelvax, Fluvirin
CPT codes: Refer to table on pages 204–205

[a]The two-dose influenza vaccine recommendations for children age 2 through 8 years may change depending on the strains in the vaccine; refer to the most current ACIP recommendations for further guidance.
[b]Persons with severe egg allergy (e.g., anaphylaxis) should be referred to a specialist for further evaluation and risk assessment; persons with hives only who are age 18–49 years may receive RIV, others should be vaccinated by a provider with allergy management experience, and patient should be observed for at least 30 minutes following vaccination.

Vaccine availability: To view the Influenza Vaccine Availability Tracking System (IVATS), go to www.preventinfluenza.org/ivats/ivats_healthcare.asp

Additional dose interchangeability: Products are interchangeable for children requiring two doses (includes LAIV when appropriate)

References

Afluria [package insert]. King of Prussia, PA: bioCSL Limited; August 2014.

Centers for Disease Control and Prevention. General recommendations on immunization: recommendations of the Advisory Committee on Immunization Practices (ACIP). *MMWR Recomm Rep.* 2011;60(RR-2):1–60.

Centers for Disease Control and Prevention. Prevention and control of influenza with vaccines: recommendations of the Advisory Committee on Immunization Practices (ACIP)—United States, 2014–2015 influenza season. *MMWR Morb Mortal Wkly Rep.* 2014;63(32):691–7.

Fluarix [package insert]. Research Triangle Park, NC: GlaxoSmithKline; June 2014.

Fluarix Quadrivalent [package insert]. Research Triangle Park, NC: GlaxoSmithKline; June 2014.

FluBlok [package insert]. Meriden, CT: Protein Sciences; October 2014.

Flucelvax [package insert]. Cambridge, MA: Novartis Vaccines and Diagnostics, Inc.; March 2014.

FluLaval [package insert]. Research Triangle Park, NC: GlaxoSmithKline; May 2014.

FluLaval Quadrivalent [package insert]. Research Triangle Park, NC: GlaxoSmithKline; May 2014.

Fluvirin [package insert]. Cambridge, MA: Novartis Vaccines and Diagnostics, Inc.; February 2014.

Fluzone [package insert]. Swiftwater, PA: Sanofi Pasteur; June 2014.

Fluzone High-Dose [package insert]. Swiftwater, PA: Sanofi Pasteur; June 2014.

Fluzone Intradermal [package insert]. Swiftwater, PA: Sanofi Pasteur; June 2014.

Fluzone Quadrivalent [package insert]. Swiftwater, PA: Sanofi Pasteur; June 2014.

Immunization Action Coalition. Guide to contraindications and precautions to commonly used vaccines. www.immunize.org/catg.d/p3072a.pdf. Accessed October 13, 2014.

Immunization Action Coalition. Influenza vaccine products for the 2014–2015 influenza season. www.immunize.org/catg.d/p4072.pdf. Accessed January 18, 2015.

2014–2015 Seasonal Influenza Vaccines

Trade name and type	Manufacturer	Age indications	Product specifications	CPT code
Afluria (IIV3)	bioCSL	≥9 years	0.5 mL prefilled syringe	90656
		≥9 years (or 18-64 via jet injector)	5 mL multi-dose vial—discard after 28 days of initial use	90658
Fluarix (IIV4)	GlaxoSmithKline	≥3 years	0.5 mL prefilled syringe	90686
Fluarix (IIV3)				90656
FluBlok (RIV3)	Protein Sciences	≥18 years	0.5 mL single-dose vial	90673
Flucelvax (ccIIV3)	Novartis	≥18 years	0.5 mL prefilled syringe—tip cap may contain latex	90661
FluLaval (IIV4)	ID Biomedical	≥3 years	0.5 mL prefilled syringe	90686
			5 mL multi-dose vial—discard after 28 days of initial use	90688
FluLaval (IIV3)	ID Biomedical	≥3 years	0.5 mL prefilled syringe	90656
			5 mL multi-dose vial—discard after 28 days of initial use	90658

Fluvirin (IIV3)	Novartis	≥4 years	0.5 mL prefilled syringe—tip cap may contain latex	90656
			5 mL multi-dose vial—do not use past expiration date on vial	90658
Fluzone (IIV4)	Sanofi Pasteur	6–35 months	0.25 mL prefilled syringe	90685
		≥3 years	0.5 mL prefilled syringe	90686
		≥3 years	0.5 mL single-dose vial	90686
		≥6 months	5 mL multi-dose vial—do not use past expiration date on vial	90687
Fluzone (IIV3)	Sanofi Pasteur	≥3 years	0.5 mL prefilled syringe	90656
		≥6 months	5 mL multi-dose vial—do not use past expiration date on vial	90657
Fluzone High-Dose (IIV3)	Sanofi Pasteur	≥65 years	0.5 mL prefilled syringe	90662
Fluzone Intradermal (IIV3)	Sanofi Pasteur	18–64 years	0.1 mL prefilled microinjection system	90654

IIV3 = inactivated influenza vaccine, trivalent
IIV4 = inactivated influenza vaccine, quadrivalent
RIV3 = recombinant influenza vaccine, trivalent
ccIIV3 = inactivated influenza vaccine, trivalent, cell culture-based

Live Attenuated Influenza Vaccine (LAIV)

Vaccine type: Live, quadrivalent
Age indications: 2 through 49 years[a]
Preparation: N/A
Storage: Store at 2°C–8°C (35°F–46°F); do not freeze
Shelf life once reconstituted: N/A
Volume and route: 0.2 mL intranasally (0.1 mL—1 spray—in each nostril)
Dosing schedule: 2 through 8 years—One or two doses,[b] 28 days apart; ≥9 years—annual
Contraindications: Severe allergic reaction to previous dose or vaccine component (e.g., eggs,[c] gentamicin, gelatin, arginine); patients <2 or ≥50 years of age; patients with asthma; children less than 5 years of age with recurrent wheezing; patients with chronic medical conditions; pregnancy; immunodeficiency; children or adolescents receiving long-term aspirin therapy; persons in close contact with severely immunosuppressed patients who are hospitalized or receiving care in a protected environment
Precautions: Moderate or severe acute illness with or without fever; history of Guillain-Barré syndrome within 6 weeks of a prior influenza vaccination
Drug interactions: Influenza antiviral agents—Do not administer vaccine until 48 hours after antiviral use is discontinued. Do not administer antiviral agents until 2 weeks after vaccine administration unless medically necessary.
CPT code: 90660

[a]LAIV is the preferred influenza vaccine for children age 2 through 8 years; if LAIV is unavailable, vaccinate this age group with the inactivated influenza vaccine (IIV).
[b]The two-dose influenza vaccine recommendations for children age 2 through 8 years may change depending on the strains in the vaccine; refer to the most current ACIP recommendations for further guidance.
[c]Studies involving egg allergy and influenza vaccination are limited to inactivated influenza vaccine (IIV); consider the use of IIV for persons with egg allergy, and follow current ACIP recommendations.

Trade name: FluMist
Manufacturer: MedImmune
Product specifications: Prefilled sprayer (10 per package)

Vaccine availability: To view the Influenza Vaccine Availability Tracking System (IVATS), go to www.preventinfluenza.org/ivats/ivats_healthcare.asp

Additional dose interchangeability: N/A

References

Centers for Disease Control and Prevention. General recommendations on immunization: recommendations of the Advisory Committee on Immunization Practices (ACIP). *MMWR Recomm Rep.* 2011;60(RR-2):1–60.
Centers for Disease Control and Prevention. Prevention and control of influenza with vaccines: recommendations of the Advisory Committee on Immunization Practices (ACIP)—United States, 2014–2015 influenza season. *MMWR Morb Mortal Wkly Rep.* 2014;63(32):691–7.
FluMist [package insert]. Gaithersburg, MD: MedImmune; July 2014.
Immunization Action Coalition. Guide to contraindications and precautions to commonly used vaccines. www.immunize.org/catg.d/p3072a.pdf. Accessed October 13, 2014.

Measles, Mumps, and Rubella Virus Vaccine (MMR)

Vaccine type: Live attenuated
Age indications: ≥12 months
Preparation: Reconstitute
Storage: Store at –50°C (–58°F); do not freeze diluent; protect from light at all times; do not ship using dry ice
Shelf life once reconstituted: 8 hours when stored at 2°C–8°C (36°F–46°F)
Volume and route: 0.5 mL subcutaneously
Dosing schedule: Two doses, first dose at 12–15 months of age and second dose at 4–6 years of age
Contraindications: Severe allergic reaction to previous dose or vaccine component (e.g., gelatin, neomycin); pregnancy; immunodeficiency
Precautions: Moderate or severe acute illness with or without fever; receipt of antibody-containing blood product within the past 11 months; history of thrombocytopenia or thrombocytopenic purpura
Interactions: Tuberculin skin testing—postpone for at least 28 days if not done prior to or simultaneous with vaccine
CPT code: 90707

Trade name: M-M-R II
Manufacturer: Merck
Product specifications: Single-dose vial of lyophilized vaccine plus diluent (10 per package)
NDC: 00006-4681-00

Additional dose interchangeability: N/A

References

Centers for Disease Control and Prevention. General recommendations on immunization: recommendations of the Advisory Committee on Immunization Practices (ACIP). *MMWR Recomm Rep.* 2011;60(RR-2):1–60.

Immunization Action Coalition. Guide to contraindications and precautions to commonly used vaccines. www.immunize.org/catg.d/p3072a.pdf. Accessed October 13, 2014.

M-M-R II [package insert]. West Point, PA: Merck; June 2014.

Meningococcal Vaccine

Vaccine type: Inactivated
Age indications: Menactra (MCV4)—9 months through 55 years
Menveo (MCV4)—2 months through 55 years
Menomune (MPSV4)—2 years through adulthood (reserve for patients >55 years who have not previously received MCV4 and require only a single dose)
Preparation: Menactra (MCV4)—Shake well
Menveo (MCV4)—Reconstitute
Menomune (MPSV4)—Reconstitute
Storage: Store at 2°C–8°C (35°F–46°F); do not freeze; MCV4—protect from light
Shelf life once reconstituted: Menveo—8 hours
Menomune single-dose vial—30 minutes; Menomune multidose vial—35 days
Volume and route: Menactra (MCV4) and Menveo (MCV4)—0.5 mL IM
Menomune (MPSV4)—0.5 mL subcutaneously
Dosing schedule: Single dose of MCV4 for all adolescents age 11 through 12 years, with booster dose at age 16; refer to ACIP recommendations for those age 2 months and older with high-risk conditions
Contraindications: Severe allergic reaction to previous dose or vaccine component
Precautions: Moderate or severe acute illness with or without fever; history of Arthus-type hypersensitivity reaction following previous dose of tetanus or diphtheria-toxoid containing vaccine (including MCV4)—defer vaccination for at least 10 years; latex allergy—Menomune vials
CPT code: MCV4—90734
MPSV4—90733

Trade name: Menactra
Manufacturer: Sanofi Pasteur
Product specifications: 0.5 mL single-dose vial (5 per package)
NDC: 49281-0589-05

Trade name: Menomune
Manufacturer: Sanofi Pasteur
Product specifications: Single-dose lyophilized vaccine plus diluents; vial stoppers contain latex
NDC: 49281-0489-01 (1 per package)
Product specifications: 5 mL multidose lyophilized vaccine plus diluents; vial stoppers contain latex
NDC: 49281-0489-91 (5 per package)—Do not use past expiration date on vial

Trade name: Menveo
Manufacturer: Novartis
Product specifications: Single-dose lyophilized vaccine plus diluent (10 per package)
NDC: 46028-0208-01

Additional dose interchangeability: MCV4 products can be interchanged if absolutely necessary (if patient is >9 months of age)

References

Centers for Disease Control and Prevention. Errata: Vol. 60, No. RR-2. *MMWR Morb Mortal Wkly Rep.* 2011;60:993.

Centers for Disease Control and Prevention. General recommendations on immunization: recommendations of the Advisory Committee on Immunization Practices (ACIP). *MMWR Recomm Rep.* 2011;60(RR-2):1–60.

Centers for Disease Control and Prevention. Recommended adult immunization schedule—United States, 2014. www.cdc.gov/vaccines/schedules/hcp/adult.html. Accessed October 13, 2014.

Immunization Action Coalition. Guide to contraindications and precautions to commonly used vaccines. www.immunize.org/catg.d/p3072a.pdf. Accessed October 13, 2014.

Menactra [package insert]. Swiftwater, PA: Sanofi Pasteur; August 2014.

Menomune [package insert]. Swiftwater, PA: Sanofi Pasteur; April 2013.

Menveo [package insert]. Cambridge, MA: Novartis Vaccines and Diagnostics; August 2013.

Pneumococcal Vaccine

Vaccine type: Inactivated
Age indications: Prevnar 13 (PCV13)—≥6 weeks
Pneumovax 23 (PPSV)—≥2 years
Preparation: Prevnar 13 (PCV13)—Shake well
Pneumovax 23 (PPSV)—N/A (available as a clear, colorless solution)
Storage: Store at 2°C–8°C (35°F–46°F); do not freeze
Shelf life once reconstituted: N/A
Volume and route: Prevnar 13 (PCV13)—0.5 mL IM
Pneumovax 23 (PPSV)—0.5 mL IM or subcutaneous (IM preferred)
Dosing schedule: PCV13—Four doses routinely given at 2, 4, 6, and 12–15 months of age
Both PCV13 and PPSV23 should be routinely administered to all adults age ≥65 years[a]
PCV13 and PPSV23 are recommended for children and adults with high-risk and immunocompromising conditions—refer to ACIP for age, condition, and dosing guidance
Contraindications: Severe allergic reaction to previous dose or vaccine component
Precautions: Moderate or severe acute illness with or without fever
Drug interactions: Although the manufacturer states concurrent administration of Zostavax and Pneumovax-23 can result in reduced immunogenicity of Zostavax, ACIP does not recommend waiting if both are needed
CPT code: Prevnar 13 (PCV13)—90670
Pneumovax 23 (PPSV)—90732

[a]If PCV13 is given first, wait 6 to 12 months to give PPSV23 (minimum interval is 8 weeks); if PPSV23 is given first, wait 1 year to give PCV13.

Trade name: Prevnar 13
Manufacturer: Wyeth
Product specifications: 0.5 mL prefilled syringe
NDC: 00005-1971-05 (1 per package); 00005-1971-02 (10 per package)

Trade name: Pneumovax 23
Manufacturer: Merck
Product specifications: 0.5 mL single-dose vial (10 per package)
NDC: 00006-4943-00
Product specifications: 0.5 mL prefilled syringe
NDC: 00006-4837-03 (10 per package)
Product specifications: 2.5 mL multidose vial (1 per package)—Do not use past expiration date on vial
NDC: 00006-4739-00

Additional dose interchangeability: N/A

References

Centers for Disease Control and Prevention. Prevention of pneumococcal disease among infants and children—use of 13-valent pneumococcal conjugate vaccine and 23-valent pneumococcal polysaccharide vaccine: recommendations of the Advisory Committee on Immunization Practices (ACIP). *MMWR Recomm Rep.* 2010;59(RR11):1–18.

Centers for Disease Control and Prevention. Use of 13-valent pneumococcal conjugate vaccine and 23-valent pneumococcal polysaccharide vaccine among adults aged ≥65 years: recommendations of the Advisory Committee on Immunization Practices (ACIP). *MMWR Recomm Rep.* 2014;63(37):822–5.

Centers for Disease Control and Prevention. Use of 13-valent pneumococcal conjugate vaccine and 23-valent pneumococcal polysaccharide vaccine for adults with immunocompromising conditions: recommendations of the Advisory Committee on Immunization Practices (ACIP). *MMWR Recomm Rep.* 2012;61(40):816–9.

Pneumovax 23 [package insert]. West Point, PA: Merck; May 2014.

Prevnar 13 [package insert]. Philadelphia, PA: Wyeth; January 2014.

Poliovirus Vaccine

Vaccine type: Inactivated
Age indications: 6 weeks through adulthood
Preparation: Shake well
Storage: Store at 2°C–8°C (35°F–46°F); do not freeze
Shelf life once reconstituted: N/A
Volume and route: 0.5 mL IM or subcutaneous
Dosing schedule: Three doses given at 2 months, 4 months, and 6–18 months of age and booster at 4–6 years of age
Contraindications: Severe allergic reaction to previous dose or vaccine component (e.g., neomycin, polymixin B, streptomycin)
Precautions: Moderate or severe acute illness with or without fever; pregnancy; latex allergy—prefilled syringe
CPT code: 90713

Trade name: IPOL
Manufacturer: Sanofi Pasteur
Product specifications: 0.5 mL prefilled syringe
NDC: 49281-0860-88 (1 per package); 49281-0860-55 (10 per package)
Product specifications: 5 mL multidose vial—Do not use past expiration date on vial
NDC: 49281-0860-78 (1 per package); 49281-0860-10 (10 per package)

Additional dose interchangeability: N/A

References

Centers for Disease Control and Prevention. General recommendations on immunization: recommendations of the Advisory Committee on Immunization Practices (ACIP). *MMWR Recomm Rep.* 2011;60(RR-2):1–60.

Immunization Action Coalition. Guide to contraindications and precautions to commonly used vaccines. www.immunize.org/catg.d/p3072a.pdf. Accessed October 13, 2014.

IPOL [package insert]. Swiftwater, PA: Sanofi Pasteur; May 2013.

Rotavirus Vaccine

Vaccine type: Live attenuated
Age indications: Rotarix—6 weeks to 24 weeks
RotaTeq—6 weeks to 32 weeks
Preparation: Rotarix—Reconstitute
RotaTeq—N/A (available as a solution)
Storage: Store at 2°C–8°C (35°F–46°F); do not freeze; protect from light
Shelf life once reconstituted: Rotarix—24 hours
Volume and route: Rotarix—1 mL given orally
RotaTeq—2 mL given orally
Dosing schedule: Rotarix—Two doses given at 2 and 4 months of age
RotaTeq—Three doses given at 2, 4, and 6 months of age
Do not initiate vaccination for infants age 15 weeks or older; maximum age for final dose is 8 months
Contraindications: Severe allergic reaction to previous dose or vaccine component; history of gastrointestinal tract congenital malformation; history of intussusception; severe combined immunodeficiency (SCID); latex allergy—Rotarix applicator
Precautions: Moderate or severe acute illness with or without fever; acute, moderate, or severe gastroenteritis; diarrhea or vomiting; immunosuppression; receipt of antibody-containing blood product within previous 6 weeks; chronic gastrointestinal disease; spina bifida; bladder exstrophy
CPT code: Rotarix—90681
RotaTeq—90680

Trade name: Rotarix
Manufacturer: GlaxoSmithKline
Product specifications: Oral applicator with diluent and transfer adapter (tip cap may contain latex)
NDC: 58160-0854-52 (10 per package)

Trade name: RotaTeq
Manufacturer: Merck
Product specifications: Single-dose tube
NDC: 00006-4047-41 (10 per package); 00006-4047-20 (25 per package)

Additional dose interchangeability: Products may be interchanged if absolutely necessary; 3 doses must be given

References

Centers for Disease Control and Prevention. General recommendations on immunization: recommendations of the Advisory Committee on Immunization Practices (ACIP). *MMWR Recomm Rep.* 2011;60(RR-2):1–64.

Centers for Disease Control and Prevention. Recommended immunization schedule for persons age 0 through 18 years—United States, 2014. www.cdc.gov/vaccines/schedules/hcp/imz/child-adolescent.html. Accessed October 13, 2014.

Immunization Action Coalition. Guide to contraindications and precautions to commonly used vaccines. www.immunize.org/catg.d/p3072a.pdf. Accessed October 13, 2014.

Rotarix [package insert]. Research Triangle Park, NC: GlaxoSmithKline; May 2014.

RotaTeq [package insert]. West Point, PA: Merck; June 2013.

Tetanus & Diphtheria Toxoids Adsorbed for Adult Use (Td)

Vaccine type: Inactivated
Age indications: ≥7 years
Preparation: Shake well
Storage: Store at 2°C–8°C (35°F–46°F); do not freeze
Shelf life once reconstituted: N/A
Volume and route: 0.5 mL IM
Dosing schedule: Booster is given every 10 years (refer to the product package insert and immunization schedules provided by CDC for additional dosing information)
Contraindications: Severe allergic reaction to previous dose or vaccine component
Precautions: Moderate or severe acute illness with or without fever; pregnancy; Guillain-Barré syndrome <6 weeks following previous dose of tetanus-containing vaccine; fever >39°C (103°F) or history of Arthus-type hypersensitivity reaction following previous dose of tetanus or diphtheria-toxoid containing vaccine (including MCV4)—defer vaccination for at least 10 years; latex allergy—TENIVAC prefilled syringe
CPT code: 90714 (preservative-free)

Trade name: None
Manufacturer: MassBioLogics
Product specifications: Single-dose vial (10 per package)
NDC: 14362-0111-03

Trade name: TENIVAC
Manufacturer: Sanofi Pasteur
Product specifications: Single-dose vial
NDC: 49281-0215-58 (1 per package); 49281-0215-10 (10 per package)
Product specifications: Prefilled syringe; tip cap may contain latex
NDC: 49281-0215-88 (1 per package); 49281-0215-15 (10 per package)

Additional dose interchangeability: Not specified

References

Centers for Disease Control and Prevention. Errata: Vol. 60, No. RR-2. *MMWR Morb Mortal Wkly Rep.* 2011;60:993.

Centers for Disease Control and Prevention. General recommendations on immunization: recommendations of the Advisory Committee on Immunization Practices (ACIP). *MMWR Recomm Rep.* 2011:60(RR-2);1–60.

Immunization Action Coalition. Guide to contraindications and precautions to commonly used vaccines. www.immunize.org/catg.d/p3072a.pdf. Accessed October 13, 2014.

TENIVAC [package insert]. Swiftwater, PA: Sanofi Pasteur; April 2013.

Tetanus and diphtheria toxoids adsorbed for adult use [package insert]. Boston, MA: MassBioLogics; April 2009.

Tetanus Toxoid, Reduced Diphtheria Toxoid, and Acellular Pertussis Vaccine Adsorbed (Tdap)

Vaccine type: Inactivated
Age indications: Adacel—11 through 64 years
Boostrix—≥10 years
Preparation: Shake well
Storage: Store at 2°C–8°C (35°F–46°F); do not freeze
Shelf life once reconstituted: N/A
Volume and route: 0.5 mL IM
Dosing schedule: ≥11 years—single, one-time dose, followed by a Td booster dose in 10 years; a dose of Tdap is recommended during each pregnancy (optimal timing for Tdap administration is between 27 and 36 weeks' gestation, but Tdap may be given at any time during pregnancy)
Contraindications: Severe allergic reaction to previous dose or vaccine component; encephalopathy not attributable to another identifiable cause within 7 days following previous dose of pertussis-containing vaccine
Precautions: Moderate or severe acute illness with or without fever; pregnancy; Guillain-Barré syndrome <6 weeks following previous dose of tetanus-containing vaccine; progressive or unstable neurologic disorder; history of Arthus-type hypersensitivity reaction following previous dose of tetanus or diphtheria-toxoid containing vaccine (including MCV4)—defer vaccination for at least 10 years; latex allergy—Boostrix prefilled syringe, Adacel prefilled syringe
CPT code: 90715

Trade name: Adacel
Manufacturer: Sanofi Pasteur
Product specifications: Prefilled syringe (tip cap may contain latex)
NDC: 49281-0400-88 (1 per package); 49281-0400-15 (5 per package)
Product specifications: Single-dose vial
NDC: 49281-0400-58 (1 per package); 49281-0400-05 (5 per package); 49281-0400-10 (10 per package)

Trade name: Boostrix
Manufacturer: GlaxoSmithKline
Product specifications: Single-dose vial
NDC: 58160-0842-01(1 per package); 58160-0842-11(10 per package)
Product specifications: Prefilled syringe (tip cap may contain latex)
NDC: 58160-0842-34 (1 per package); 58160-0842-52 (10 per package)

Additional dose interchangeability: Not specified

References

Adacel [package insert]. Swiftwater, PA: Sanofi Pasteur; March 2014.

Boostrix [package insert]. Research Triangle Park, NC: GlaxoSmithKline; November 2013.

Centers for Disease Control and Prevention. Errata: Vol. 60, No. RR-2. *MMWR Morb Mortal Wkly Rep.* 2011;60:993.

Centers for Disease Control and Prevention. General recommendations on immunization: recommendations of the Advisory Committee on Immunization Practices (ACIP). *MMWR Recomm Rep.* 2011:60(RR-2);1–60.

Centers for Disease Control and Prevention. Updated recommendations for use of tetanus toxoid, reduced diphtheria toxoid, and acellular pertussis vaccine (Tdap) in pregnant women—Advisory Committee on Immunization Practices (ACIP), 2012. *MMWR Morb Mortal Wkly Rep.* 2013;62(07):131–5.

Immunization Action Coalition. Guide to contraindications and precautions to commonly used vaccines. www.immunize.org/catg.d/p3072a.pdf. Accessed October 13, 2014.

Varicella Vaccine

Vaccine type: Live attenuated
Age indications: ≥12 months
Preparation: Reconstitute
Storage:[a] Store at −50°C to −15°C (−58°F to +5°F); do not freeze diluent; protect from light prior to reconstitution; do not ship using dry ice
Shelf life once reconstituted: 30 minutes
Volume and route: 0.5 mL subcutaneous
Dosing schedule: Two doses
1 to 12 years of age—second dose given at least 3 months after the first dose
≥13 years of age—second dose given 4 to 8 weeks after the first dose
Contraindications: Severe allergic reaction to previous dose or vaccine component (e.g., neomycin, gelatin); immunosuppression; active untreated tuberculosis; pregnancy
Precautions: Moderate or severe acute illness with or without fever; receipt of antibody-containing blood product within the past 11 months
Drug interactions: Antiviral medications used against herpes may reduce the effectiveness if given less than 24 hours prior to or within 14 days following vaccine; tuberculin skin testing—postpone for at least 6 weeks if not done prior to or simultaneously with vaccine
CPT code: 90716

[a]Varicella products may be stored and/or transported at 2°–8°C (36°–46°F) for up to 72 continuous hours prior to reconstitution. If vaccine stored at this temperature is not used within 72 hours, it must be discarded.

Trade name: Varivax
Manufacturer: Merck
Product specifications: Single-dose vial of lyophilized vaccine
NDC: 00006-4826-00 (1 per package plus 10 vials of diluent); 00006-4827-00 (10 per package plus 10 vials of diluent)

Additional dose interchangeability: N/A

References

Centers for Disease Control and Prevention. General recommendations on immunization: recommendations of the Advisory Committee on Immunization Practices (ACIP). *MMWR Recomm Rep.* 2011:60(RR-2);1–60.

Immunization Action Coalition. Guide to contraindications and precautions to commonly used vaccines. www.immunize.org/catg.d/p3072a.pdf. Accessed October 13, 2014.

Varivax [package insert]. West Point, PA: Merck; July 2014.

Combination Vaccine Products

Trade name: Kinrix
Components: DTaP + IPV
Manufacturer: GlaxoSmithKline
Preparation: Shake well
Storage: Store at 2°C–8°C (35°F–46°F); do not freeze
CPT code: 90696
Product specifications: Single-dose vial
NDC: 58160-0812-01 (1 per package); 58160-0812-11 (10 per package)
Product specifications: Prefilled syringe (tip cap may contain latex)
NDC: 58160-0812-43 (1 per package); 58160-0812-52 (10 per package)

Trade name: Menhibrix
Components: Meningococcal Groups C and Y + Hib
Manufacturer: GlaxoSmithKline
Preparation: Reconstitute
Storage: Store at 2°C–8°C (35°F–46°F); do not freeze
Shelf life once reconstituted: Use immediately after reconstitution
CPT code: 90644
Product specifications: Single-dose vial of lyophilized vaccine
NDC: 58160-0801-11 (10 per package plus 10 vials of diluent)

Trade name: Pediarix
Components: DTaP + Hepatitis B + IPV
Manufacturer: GlaxoSmithKline
Preparation: Shake well
Storage: Store at 2°C–8°C (35°F–46°F); do not freeze
CPT code: 90723
Product specifications: Prefilled syringe (tip cap may contain latex)
NDC: 58160-0811-43 (1 per package); 58160-0811-52 (10 per package)

Trade name: Pentacel
Components: DTaP + IPV + Hib
Manufacturer: Sanofi Pasteur
Preparation: Reconstitute
Storage: Store at 2°C–8°C (35°F–46°F); do not freeze
Shelf life once reconstituted: Use immediately after reconstitution
CPT code: 90698
Product specifications: 5 single-dose vials of DTap+IPV used to reconstitute 5 single-dose vials of lyophilized ActHIB
NDC: 49281-0510-05

Trade name: ProQuad
Components: MMR + Varicella
Manufacturer: Merck
Preparation: Reconstitute
Storage: Store at –50°C to –15°C (–58°F to +5°F); do not freeze diluent; protect from light prior to reconstitution; do not ship using dry ice; may be stored and/or transported at 2°–8°C (36°–46°F) for up to 72 continuous hours prior to reconstitution (if vaccine stored at this temperature is not used within 72 hours, it must be discarded)
Shelf life once reconstituted: 30 minutes
CPT code: 90710
Product specifications: Single-dose vial of lyophilized vaccine (10 per package) plus 10 vials of diluent
NDC: 00006-4999-00

Trade name: Twinrix
Components: Hepatitis A + Hepatitis B
Manufacturer: GlaxoSmithKline
Preparation: Shake well
Storage: Store at 2°C–8°C (35°F–46°F); do not freeze
CPT code: 90636
Product specifications: Single-dose vial
NDC: 58160-0815-01 (1 per package); 58160-0815-11 (10 per package)
Product specifications: Prefilled syringe (tip cap may contain latex)
NDC: 58160-0815-34 (1 per package); 58160-0815-52 (10 per package)

References

Kinrix [package insert]. Research Triangle Park, NC: GlaxoSmithKline; July 2014.

Menhibrix [package insert]. Research Triangle Park, NC: GlaxoSmithKline; November 2013.

Pediarix [package insert]. Research Triangle Park, NC: GlaxoSmithKline; November 2013.

Pentacel [package insert]. Swiftwater, PA: Sanofi Pasteur; October 2013.

ProQuad [package insert]. West Point, PA: Merck; March 2014.

Twinrix [package insert]. Research Triangle Park, NC: GlaxoSmithKline; December 2013.

Chapter 20

Immunization Schedules

At the beginning of each year, CDC publishes updated immunization schedules for children and adults. The schedules are designed so that providers can quickly and accurately identify which vaccinations their patients need. The left-hand column of each table lists the applicable vaccines. The various patient groups are noted across the tops of the tables. Color-coded bars are used to highlight which vaccines are recommended for each group.

In this chapter, you will find the 2015 adult and childhood immunization schedules. When new schedules are released each year, you can print the pocket-size schedules from the CDC website and insert them on the respective pages in this chapter.

To locate and print the pocket-size immunization schedules, complete the following steps:

1. Go to www.cdc.gov/vaccines.
2. Click on Immunization Schedules in the left-hand column.
3. Click on the schedule you want.
4. Select pocket size.
5. Print each schedule. The color versions are preferred for easier reading of the schedules.
6. Trim each to size and glue or tape onto the respective pages.

Two schedules for adults have been included (Figures 20.1 and 20.2). The first is based on age, and the second is categorized by medical conditions and other indications. The schedule for children and adolescents includes those age 0 through 18 years (Figure 20.3). Not included in this book is the entire catch-up schedule. If you are working with children who have started their immunizations later than recommended or are more than 1 month behind, you will need to refer to the CDC website to access the most current catch-up schedule (www.cdc.gov/vaccines/schedules/hcp/child-adolescent.html). Also available via this Web page are links to the interactive schedulers for catch-up immunizations, adolescent vaccines, and adult vaccines needed. Once you have downloaded this tool, you can use it to quickly locate any missing immunizations for the individual patient. You can also access the CDC Vaccines Schedules app from this page.

When reading the immunization schedules, you must also remember to read the footnotes. If footnotes have not been included in the pocket-size versions created by CDC, you will need to access the original schedules to review them. The footnotes include important information regarding specific vaccine recommendations and conditions. This is particularly critical in working with patients who have special vaccination needs (e.g., pregnant patients; patients with hepatitis C or chronic liver disease; patients with asplenia, HIV, and other conditions that compromise the immune system). You are bound to encounter questions or concerns from these patients, their caregivers, or other health care providers. Knowing where to find such information will be valuable. Additional information on these groups can be found in the statements from the Advisory Committee on Immunization Practices (www.cdc.gov/vaccines/hcp/acip-recs/index.html), and recommendations for immunocompromising and high-risk conditions are summarized in Chapter 16.

Figure 20.1

Recommended Adult Immunization Schedule, by Vaccine and Age Group

Recommended Adult Immunization Schedule—United States - 2015

Note: These recommendations must be read with the footnotes that follow containing number of doses, intervals between doses, and other important information.

Figure 1. Recommended adult immunization schedule, by vaccine and age group[1]

VACCINE ▼ AGE GROUP ▶	19-21 years	22-26 years	27-49 years	50-59 years	60-64 years	≥ 65 years
Influenza[*,2]	1 dose annually					
Tetanus, diphtheria, pertussis (Td/Tdap),[*,3]	Substitute 1-time dose of Tdap for Td booster; then boost with Td every 10 yrs					
Varicella[*,4]	2 doses					
Human papillomavirus (HPV) Female[*,5]	3 doses					
Human papillomavirus (HPV) Male[*,5]	3 doses					
Zoster[6]					1 dose	
Measles, mumps, rubella (MMR)[*,7]	1 or 2 doses					
Pneumococcal 13-valent conjugate (PCV13)[*,8]	1-time dose					
Pneumococcal polysaccharide (PPSV23)[8]	1 or 2 doses					1 dose
Meningococcal[*,9]	1 or more doses					
Hepatitis A[*,10]	2 doses					
Hepatitis B[*,11]	3 doses					
Haemophilus influenzae type b (Hib)[*,12]	1 or 3 doses					

*Covered by the Vaccine Injury Compensation Program

- For all persons in this category who meet the age requirements and who lack documentation of vaccination or have no evidence of previous infection; zoster vaccine recommended regardless of prior episode of zoster
- Recommended if some other risk factor is present (e.g., on the basis of medical, occupational, lifestyle, or other indication)
- No recommendation

Report all clinically significant postvaccination reactions to the Vaccine Adverse Event Reporting System (VAERS). Reporting forms and instructions on filing a VAERS report are available at www.vaers.hhs.gov or by telephone, 800-822-7967.
Information on how to file a Vaccine Injury Compensation Program claim is available at www.hrsa.gov/vaccinecompensation or by telephone, 800-338-2382. To file a claim for vaccine injury, contact the U.S. Court of Federal Claims, 717 Madison Place, N.W., Washington, D.C. 20005; telephone, 202-357-6400.
Additional information about the vaccines in this schedule, extent of available data, and contraindications for vaccination is also available at www.cdc.gov/vaccines or from the CDC-INFO Contact Center at 800-CDC-INFO (800-232-4636) in English and Spanish, 8:00 a.m. - 8:00 p.m. Eastern Time, Monday - Friday, excluding holidays.
Use of trade names and commercial sources is for identification only and does not imply endorsement by the U.S. Department of Health and Human Services.

The recommendations in this schedule were approved by the Centers for Disease Control and Prevention's (CDC) Advisory Committee on Immunization Practices (ACIP), the American Academy of Family Physicians (AAFP), the American College of Physicians (ACP), American College of Obstetricians and Gynecologists (ACOG) and American College of Nurse-Midwives (ACNM).

Figure 20.2

Recommended Adult Immunization Schedule, Based on Indication

Figure 2. Vaccines that might be indicated for adults based on medical and other indications[1]

VACCINE ▼ INDICATION ▶	Pregnancy	Immunocompromising conditions (excluding human immunodeficiency virus [HIV]) [4,6,7,8,13]	HIV infection CD4+ T lymphocyte count [4,6,7,8,13] < 200 cells/μL	HIV infection CD4+ T lymphocyte count ≥ 200 cells/μL	Men who have sex with men (MSM)	Kidney failure, end-stage renal disease, receipt of hemodialysis	Heart disease, chronic lung disease, chronic alcoholism	Asplenia (including elective splenectomy and persistent complement component deficiencies) [8,12]	Chronic liver disease	Diabetes	Healthcare personnel
Influenza*[,2]	1 dose IIV annually				1 dose IIV or LAIV annually	1 dose IIV annually					1 dose IIV or LAIV annually
Tetanus, diphtheria, pertussis (Td/Tdap)*[,3]	1 dose Tdap each pregnancy	Substitute 1-time dose of Tdap for Td booster; then boost with Td every 10 yrs									
Varicella*[,4]	Contraindicated			2 doses							
Human papillomavirus (HPV) Female*[,5]		3 doses through age 26 yrs				3 doses through age 26 yrs					
Human papillomavirus (HPV) Male*[,5]		3 doses through age 26yrs				3 doses through age 21 yrs					
Zoster[6]	Contraindicated				1 dose						
Measles, mumps, rubella (MMR)*[,7]	Contraindicated			1 or 2 doses							
Pneumococcal 13-valent conjugate (PCV13)*[,8]		1 dose									
Pneumococcal polysaccharide (PPSV23)[8]	1 or 2 doses										
Meningococcal*[,9]	1 or more doses										
Hepatitis A*[,10]	2 doses										
Hepatitis B*[,11]	3 doses										
Haemophilus influenzae type b (Hib)*[,12]		post-HSCT recipients only	1 or 3 doses								

*Covered by the Vaccine Injury Compensation Program

- (light shading) For all persons in this category who meet the age requirements and who lack documentation of vaccination or have no evidence of previous infection; zoster vaccine recommended regardless of prior episode of zoster
- (dark shading) Recommended if some other risk factor is present (e.g., on the basis of medical, occupational, lifestyle, or other indications)
- (no shading) No recommendation

U.S. Department of Health and Human Services
Centers for Disease Control and Prevention

These schedules indicate the recommended age groups and medical indications for which administration of currently licensed vaccines is commonly recommended for adults ages 19 years and older, as of February 1, 2015. For all vaccines being recommended on the Adult Immunization Schedule: a vaccine series does not need to be restarted, regardless of the time that has elapsed between doses. Licensed combination vaccines may be used whenever any components of the combination are indicated and when the vaccine's other components are not contraindicated. For detailed recommendations on all vaccines, including those used primarily for travelers or that are issued during the year, consult the manufacturers' package inserts and the complete statements from the Advisory Committee on Immunization Practices (www.cdc.gov/vaccines/hcp/acip-recs/index.html). Use of trade names and commercial sources is for identification only and does not imply endorsement by the U.S. Department of Health and Human Services.

Footnotes for Figures 20.1 and 20.2, Recommended Adult Immunization Schedule—United States, 2015

1. **Additional information**
   - Additional guidance for the use of the vaccines described in this supplement is available at www.cdc.gov/vaccines/hcp/acip-recs/index.html.
   - Information on vaccination recommendations when vaccination status is unknown and other general immunization information can be found in the General Recommendations on Immunization at www.cdc.gov/mmwr/preview/mmwrhtml/rr6002a1.htm.
   - Information on travel vaccine requirements and recommendations (e.g., for hepatitis A and B, meningococcal, and other vaccines) is available at wwwnc.cdc.gov/travel/destinations/list.
   - Additional information and resources regarding vaccination of pregnant women can be found at www.cdc.gov/vaccines/adults/rec-vac/pregnant.html.
2. **Influenza vaccination**
   - Annual vaccination against influenza is recommended for all persons aged 6 months or older.
   - Persons aged 6 months or older, including pregnant women and persons with hives-only allergy to eggs can receive the inactivated influenza vaccine (IIV). An age-appropriate IIV formulation should be used.
   - Adults aged 18 years or older can receive the recombinant influenza vaccine (RIV) (FluBlok). RIV does not contain any egg protein and can be given to age-appropriate persons with egg allergy of any severity.
   - Healthy, nonpregnant persons aged 2 to 49 years without high-risk medical conditions can receive either intranasally administered live, attenuated influenza vaccine (LAIV) (FluMist) or IIV.
   - Health care personnel who care for severely immunocompromised persons who require care in a protected environment should receive IIV or RIV; health care personnel who receive LAIV should avoid providing care for severely immunosuppressed persons for 7 days after vaccination.
   - The intramuscularly or intradermally administered IIV are options for adults aged 18 through 64 years.
   - Adults aged 65 years or older can receive the standard-dose IIV or the high-dose IIV (Fluzone High-Dose).
   - A list of currently available influenza vaccines can be found at www.cdc.gov/flu/protect/vaccine/vaccines.htm.
3. **Tetanus, diphtheria, and acellular pertussis (Td/Tdap) vaccination**
   - Administer 1 dose of Tdap vaccine to pregnant women during each pregnancy (preferably during 27 to 36 weeks' gestation) regardless of interval since prior Td or Tdap vaccination.
   - Persons aged 11 years or older who have not received Tdap vaccine or for whom vaccine status is unknown should receive a dose of Tdap followed by tetanus and diphtheria toxoids (Td) booster doses every 10 years thereafter. Tdap can be administered regardless of interval since the most recent tetanus or diphtheria-toxoid containing vaccine.
   - Adults with an unknown or incomplete history of completing a 3-dose primary vaccination series with Td-containing vaccines should begin or complete a primary vaccination series including a Tdap dose.

continued on page 232

Footnotes for Figures 20.1 and 20.2, *continued from page 231*

- For unvaccinated adults, administer the first 2 doses at least 4 weeks apart and the third dose 6 to 12 months after the second.
- For incompletely vaccinated (i.e., less than 3 doses) adults, administer remaining doses.
- Refer to the ACIP statement for recommendations for administering Td/Tdap as prophylaxis in wound management (see footnote 1).

4. **Varicella vaccination**
   - All adults without evidence of immunity to varicella (as defined below) should receive 2 doses of single-antigen varicella vaccine or a second dose if they have received only 1 dose.
   - Vaccination should be emphasized for those who have close contact with persons at high risk for severe disease (e.g., health care personnel and family contacts of persons with immunocompromising conditions) or are at high risk for exposure or transmission (e.g., teachers; child care employees; residents and staff members of institutional settings, including correctional institutions; college students; military personnel; adolescents and adults living in households with children; nonpregnant women of childbearing age; and international travelers).
   - Pregnant women should be assessed for evidence of varicella immunity. Women who do not have evidence of immunity should receive the first dose of varicella vaccine upon completion or termination of pregnancy and before discharge from the health care facility. The second dose should be administered 4 to 8 weeks after the first dose.
   - Evidence of immunity to varicella in adults includes any of the following:
     — documentation of 2 doses of varicella vaccine at least 4 weeks apart;
     — U.S.-born before 1980, except health care personnel and pregnant women;
     — history of varicella based on diagnosis or verification of varicella disease by a health care provider;
     — history of herpes zoster based on diagnosis or verification of herpes zoster disease by a health care provider; or
     — laboratory evidence of immunity or laboratory confirmation of disease.

5. **Human papillomavirus (HPV) vaccination**
   - Two vaccines are licensed for use in females, bivalent HPV vaccine (HPV2) and quadrivalent HPV vaccine (HPV4), and one HPV vaccine for use in males (HPV4).
   - For females, either HPV4 or HPV2 is recommended in a 3-dose series for routine vaccination at age 11 or 12 years and for those aged 13 through 26 years, if not previously vaccinated.
   - For males, HPV4 is recommended in a 3-dose series for routine vaccination at age 11 or 12 years and for those aged 13 through 21 years, if not previously vaccinated. Males aged 22 through 26 years may be vaccinated.
   - HPV4 is recommended for men who have sex with men through age 26 years for those who did not get any or all doses when they were younger.
   - Vaccination is recommended for immunocompromised persons (including those with HIV infection) through age 26 years for those who did not get any or all doses when they were younger.
   - A complete series for either HPV4 or HPV2 consists of 3 doses. The second dose should be administered 4 to 8 weeks (minimum interval of 4 weeks) after the first dose; the third dose should be administered 24 weeks after the first dose and 16 weeks after the second dose (minimum interval of at least 12 weeks).

- HPV vaccines are not recommended for use in pregnant women. However, pregnancy testing is not needed before vaccination. If a woman is found to be pregnant after initiating the vaccination series, no intervention is needed; the remainder of the 3-dose series should be delayed until completion or termination of pregnancy.

6. **Zoster vaccination**
   - A single dose of zoster vaccine is recommended for adults aged 60 years or older regardless of whether they report a prior episode of herpes zoster. Although the vaccine is licensed by the U.S. Food and Drug Administration for use among and can be administered to persons aged 50 years or older, ACIP recommends that vaccination begin at age 60 years.
   - Persons aged 60 years or older with chronic medical conditions may be vaccinated unless their condition constitutes a contraindication, such as pregnancy or severe immunodeficiency.

7. **Measles, mumps, rubella (MMR) vaccination**
   - Adults born before 1957 are generally considered immune to measles and mumps. All adults born in 1957 or later should have documentation of 1 or more doses of MMR vaccine unless they have a medical contraindication to the vaccine or laboratory evidence of immunity to each of the three diseases. Documentation of provider-diagnosed disease is not considered acceptable evidence of immunity for measles, mumps, or rubella.

   Measles component:
   - A routine second dose of MMR vaccine, administered a minimum of 28 days after the first dose, is recommended for adults who:
     — are students in postsecondary educational institutions,
     — work in a health care facility, or
     — plan to travel internationally.
   - Persons who received inactivated (killed) measles vaccine or measles vaccine of unknown type during 1963–1967 should be revaccinated with 2 doses of MMR vaccine.

   Mumps component:
   - A routine second dose of MMR vaccine, administered a minimum of 28 days after the first dose, is recommended for adults who:
     — are students in a postsecondary educational institution,
     — work in a health care facility, or
     — plan to travel internationally.
   - Persons vaccinated before 1979 with either killed mumps vaccine or mumps vaccine of unknown type who are at high risk for mumps infection (e.g., persons who are working in a health care facility) should be considered for revaccination with 2 doses of MMR vaccine.

   Rubella component:
   - For women of childbearing age, regardless of birth year, rubella immunity should be determined. If there is no evidence of immunity, women who are not pregnant should be vaccinated. Pregnant women who do not have evidence of immunity should receive MMR vaccine upon completion or termination of pregnancy and before discharge from the health care facility.

continued on page 234

Footnotes for Figures 20.1 and 20.2, *continued from page 233*

Health care personnel born before 1957:

- For unvaccinated health care personnel born before 1957 who lack laboratory evidence of measles, mumps, and/or rubella immunity or laboratory confirmation of disease, health care facilities should consider vaccinating personnel with 2 doses of MMR vaccine at the appropriate interval for measles and mumps or 1 dose of MMR vaccine for rubella.

8. **Pneumococcal (13-valent pneumococcal conjugate vaccine [PCV13] and 23-valent pneumococcal polysaccharide vaccine [PPSV23]) vaccination**

- General information
  - — When indicated, only a single dose of PCV13 is recommended for adults.
  - — No additional dose of PPSV23 is indicated for adults vaccinated with PPSV23 at or after age 65 years.
  - — When both PCV13 and PPSV23 are indicated, PCV13 should be administered first; PCV13 and PPSV23 should not be administered during the same visit.
  - — When indicated, PCV13 and PPSV23 should be administered to adults whose pneumococcal vaccination history is incomplete or unknown.
- Adults aged 65 years or older who
  - — Have not received PCV13 or PPSV23: Administer PCV13 followed by PPSV23 in 6 to 12 months.
  - — Have not received PCV13 but have received a dose of PPSV23 at age 65 years or older: Administer PCV13 at least 1 year after the dose of PPSV23 received at age 65 years or older.
  - — Have not received PCV13 but have received 1 or more doses of PPSV23 before age 65: Administer PCV13 at least 1 year after the most recent dose of PPSV23; administer a dose of PPSV23 6 to 12 months after PCV13, or as soon as possible if this time window has passed, and at least 5 years after the most recent dose of PPSV23.
  - — Have received PCV13 but not PPSV23 before age 65 years: Administer PPSV23 6 to 12 months after PCV13 or as soon as possible if this time window has passed.
  - — Have received PCV13 and 1 or more doses of PPSV23 before age 65 years: Administer PPSV23 6 to 12 months after PCV13, or as soon as possible if this time window has passed, and at least 5 years after the most recent dose of PPSV23.
- Adults aged 19 through 64 years with immunocompromising conditions or anatomical or functional asplenia (defined below) who
  - — Have not received PCV13 or PPSV23: Administer PCV13 followed by PPSV23 at least 8 weeks after PCV13; administer a second dose of PPSV23 at least 5 years after the first dose of PPSV23.
  - — Have not received PCV13 but have received 1 dose of PPSV23: Administer PCV13 at least 1 year after the PPSV23; administer a second dose of PPSV23 at least 8 weeks after PCV13 and at least 5 years after the first dose of PPSV23.
  - — Have not received PCV13 but have received 2 doses of PPSV23: Administer PCV13 at least 1 year after the most recent dose of PPSV23.
  - — Have received PCV13 but not PPSV23: Administer PPSV23 at least 8 weeks after PCV13; administer a second dose of PPSV23 at least 5 years after the first dose of PPSV23.
  - — Have received PCV13 and 1 dose of PPSV23: Administer a second dose of PPSV23 at least 5 years after the first dose of PPSV23.

- Adults aged 19 through 64 years with cerebrospinal fluid leaks or cochlear implants: Administer PCV13 followed by PPSV23 at least 8 weeks after PCV13.
- Adults aged 19 through 64 years with chronic heart disease (including congestive heart failure and cardiomyopathies, excluding hypertension), chronic lung disease (including chronic obstructive lung disease, emphysema, and asthma), chronic liver disease (including cirrhosis), alcoholism, or diabetes mellitus: Administer PPSV23.
- Adults aged 19 through 64 years who smoke cigarettes or reside in nursing home or long-term care facilities: Administer PPSV23.
- Routine pneumococcal vaccination is not recommended for American Indian/Alaska Native or other adults unless they have the indications as above; however, public health authorities may consider recommending the use of pneumococcal vaccines for American Indians/Alaska Natives or other adults who live in areas with increased risk for invasive pneumococcal disease.
- Immunocompromising conditions that are indications for pneumococcal vaccination are: Congenital or acquired immunodeficiency (including B- or T-lymphocyte deficiency, complement deficiencies, and phagocytic disorders excluding chronic granulomatous disease), HIV infection, chronic renal failure, nephrotic syndrome, leukemia, lymphoma, Hodgkin disease, generalized malignancy, multiple myeloma, solid organ transplant, and iatrogenic immunosuppression (including long-term systemic corticosteroids and radiation therapy).
- Anatomical or functional asplenia that are indications for pneumococcal vaccination are: Sickle cell disease and other hemoglobinopathies, congenital or acquired asplenia, splenic dysfunction, and splenectomy. Administer pneumococcal vaccines at least 2 weeks before immunosuppressive therapy or an elective splenectomy, and as soon as possible to adults who are newly diagnosed with asymptomatic or symptomatic HIV infection.

9. Meningococcal vaccination

- Administer 2 doses of quadrivalent meningococcal conjugate vaccine (MenACWY [Menactra, Menveo]) at least 2 months apart to adults of all ages with anatomical or functional asplenia or persistent complement component deficiencies. HIV infection is not an indication for routine vaccination with MenACWY. If an HIV-infected person of any age is vaccinated, 2 doses of MenACWY should be administered at least 2 months apart.
- Administer a single dose of meningococcal vaccine to microbiologists routinely exposed to isolates of Neisseria meningitidis, military recruits, persons at risk during an outbreak attributable to a vaccine serogroup, and persons who travel to or live in countries in which meningococcal disease is hyperendemic or epidemic.
- First-year college students up through age 21 years who are living in residence halls should be vaccinated if they have not received a dose on or after their 16th birthday.
- MenACWY is preferred for adults with any of the preceding indications who are aged 55 years or younger as well as for adults aged 56 years or older who a) were vaccinated previously with MenACWY and are recommended for revaccination, or b) for whom multiple doses are anticipated. Meningococcal polysaccharide vaccine (MPSV4 [Menomune]) is preferred for adults aged 56 years or older who have not received MenACWY previously and who require a single dose only (e.g., travelers).
- Revaccination with MenACWY every 5 years is recommended for adults previously vaccinated with MenACWY or MPSV4 who remain at increased risk for infection (e.g., adults with anatomical or functional asplenia, persistent complement component deficiencies, or microbiologists).

10. Hepatitis A vaccination

- Vaccinate any person seeking protection from hepatitis A virus (HAV) infection and persons with any of the following indications:
  — men who have sex with men and persons who use injection or noninjection illicit drugs;

continued on page 236

Footnotes for Figures 20.1 and 20.2, *continued from page 235*

- — persons working with HAV-infected primates or with HAV in a research laboratory setting;
- — persons with chronic liver disease and persons who receive clotting factor concentrates;
- — persons traveling to or working in countries that have high or intermediate endemicity of hepatitis A; and
- — unvaccinated persons who anticipate close personal contact (e.g., household or regular babysitting) with an international adoptee during the first 60 days after arrival in the United States from a country with high or intermediate endemicity. (See footnote 1 for more information on travel recommendations.) The first dose of the 2-dose hepatitis A vaccine series should be administered as soon as adoption is planned, ideally 2 or more weeks before the arrival of the adoptee.

- Single-antigen vaccine formulations should be administered in a 2-dose schedule at either 0 and 6 to 12 months (Havrix), or 0 and 6 to 18 months (Vaqta). If the combined hepatitis A and hepatitis B vaccine (Twinrix) is used, administer 3 doses at 0, 1, and 6 months; alternatively, a 4-dose schedule may be used, administered on days 0, 7, and 21 to 30 followed by a booster dose at month 12.

11. Hepatitis B vaccination

- Vaccinate persons with any of the following indications and any person seeking protection from hepatitis B virus (HBV) infection:
  - — sexually active persons who are not in a long-term, mutually monogamous relationship (e.g., persons with more than 1 sex partner during the previous 6 months); persons seeking evaluation or treatment for a sexually transmitted disease (STD); current or recent injection drug users; and men who have sex with men;
  - — health care personnel and public safety workers who are potentially exposed to blood or other infectious body fluids;
  - — persons with diabetes who are younger than age 60 years as soon as feasible after diagnosis; persons with diabetes who are age 60 years or older at the discretion of the treating clinician based on the likelihood of acquiring HBV infection, including the risk posed by an increased need for assisted blood glucose monitoring in long-term care facilities, the likelihood of experiencing chronic sequelae if infected with HBV, and the likelihood of immune response to vaccination;
  - — persons with end-stage renal disease, including patients receiving hemodialysis, persons with HIV infection, and persons with chronic liver disease;
  - — household contacts and sex partners of hepatitis B surface antigen–positive persons, clients and staff members of institutions for persons with developmental disabilities, and international travelers to countries with high or intermediate prevalence of chronic HBV infection; and
  - — all adults in the following settings: STD treatment facilities, HIV testing and treatment facilities, facilities providing drug abuse treatment and prevention services, health care settings targeting services to injection drug users or men who have sex with men, correctional facilities, end-stage renal disease programs and facilities for chronic hemodialysis patients, and institutions and nonresidential day care facilities for persons with developmental disabilities.
- Administer missing doses to complete a 3-dose series of hepatitis B vaccine to those persons not vaccinated or not completely vaccinated. The second dose should be administered 1 month after the first dose; the third dose should be given at least 2 months after the second dose (and at least 4 months after the first dose). If the combined hepatitis A and hepatitis B vaccine (Twinrix) is used, give 3 doses at 0, 1, and 6 months; alternatively, a 4-dose Twinrix schedule, administered on days 0, 7, and 21 to 30 followed by a booster dose at month 12 may be used.
- Adult patients receiving hemodialysis or with other immunocompromising conditions should receive 1 dose of 40 mcg/mL (Recombivax HB) administered on a 3-dose schedule at 0, 1, and 6 months or 2 doses of 20 mcg/mL (Engerix-B) administered simultaneously on a 4-dose schedule at 0, 1, 2, and 6 months.

12. **Haemophilus influenzae type b (Hib) vaccination**
    - One dose of Hib vaccine should be administered to persons who have anatomical or functional asplenia or sickle cell disease or are undergoing elective splenectomy if they have not previously received Hib vaccine. Hib vaccination 14 or more days before splenectomy is suggested.
    - Recipients of a hematopoietic stem cell transplant (HSCT) should be vaccinated with a 3-dose regimen 6 to 12 months after a successful transplant, regardless of vaccination history; at least 4 weeks should separate doses.
    - Hib vaccine is not recommended for adults with HIV infection since their risk for Hib infection is low.
13. **Immunocompromising conditions**
    - Inactivated vaccines generally are acceptable (e.g., pneumococcal, meningococcal, and inactivated influenza vaccine) and live vaccines generally are avoided in persons with immune deficiencies or immunocompromising conditions. Information on specific conditions is available at www.cdc.gov/vaccines/hcp/acip-recs/index.html.

Figure 20.3

Recommended Immunization Schedule for Persons Aged 0 through 18 Years—United States, 2015

Vaccine	Birth	1 mo	2 mos	4 mos	6 mos	9 mos	12 mos	15 mos	18 mos	19–23 mos	2-3 yrs	4-6 yrs	7-10 yrs	11-12 yrs	13–15 yrs	16–18 yrs
Hepatitis B[1] (HepB)	1st dose	←------ 2nd dose ------→			←------ 3rd dose ------→											
Rotavirus[2] (RV) RV1 (2-dose series); RV5 (3-dose series)			1st dose	2nd dose	See footnote 2											
Diphtheria, tetanus, & acellular pertussis[3] (DTaP: <7 yrs)			1st dose	2nd dose	3rd dose			←------ 4th dose ------→				5th dose				
Tetanus, diphtheria, & acellular pertussis[4] (Tdap: ≥7 yrs)														(Tdap)		
Haemophilus influenzae type b[5] (Hib)			1st dose	2nd dose	See footnote 5		←--- 3rd or 4th dose, See footnote 5 ---→									
Pneumococcal conjugate[6] (PCV13)			1st dose	2nd dose	3rd dose		←------ 4th dose ------→									
Pneumococcal polysaccharide[6] (PPSV23)																
Inactivated poliovirus[7] (IPV: <18 yrs)			1st dose	2nd dose	←------ 3rd dose ------→							4th dose				
Influenza[8] (IIV; LAIV) 2 doses for some: See footnote 8					Annual vaccination (IIV only) 1 or 2 doses						Annual vaccination (LAIV or IIV) 1 or 2 doses		Annual vaccination (LAIV or IIV) 1 dose only			
Measles, mumps, rubella[9] (MMR)					See footnote 9		←------ 1st dose ------→					2nd dose				
Varicella[10] (VAR)							←------ 1st dose ------→					2nd dose				
Hepatitis A[11] (HepA)							←------ 2-dose series, See footnote 11 ------→									
Human papillomavirus[12] (HPV2: females only; HPV4: males and females)														(3-dose series)		
Meningococcal[13] (Hib-MenCY ≥ 6 weeks; MenACWY-D ≥9 mos; MenACWY-CRM ≥ 2 mos)			See footnote 13											1st dose		Booster

Range of recommended ages for all children

Range of recommended ages for catch-up immunization

Range of recommended ages for certain high-risk groups

Range of recommended ages during which catch-up is encouraged and for certain high-risk groups

Not routinely recommended

This schedule includes recommendations in effect as of January 1, 2015. Any dose not administered at the recommended age should be administered at a subsequent visit, when indicated and feasible. The use of a combination vaccine generally is preferred over separate injections of its equivalent component vaccines. Vaccination providers should consult the relevant Advisory Committee on Immunization Practices (ACIP) statement for detailed recommendations, available online at http://www.cdc.gov/vaccines/hcp/acip-recs/index.html. Clinically significant adverse events that follow vaccination should be reported to the Vaccine Adverse Event Reporting System (VAERS) online (http://www.vaers.hhs.gov) or by telephone (800-822-7967). Suspected cases of vaccine-preventable diseases should be reported to the state or local health department. Additional information, including precautions and contraindications for vaccination, is available from CDC online (http://www.cdc.gov/vaccines/recs/vac-admin/contraindications.htm) or by telephone (800-CDC-INFO [800-232-4636]).

This schedule is approved by the Advisory Committee on Immunization Practices (http//www.cdc.gov/vaccines/acip), the American Academy of Pediatrics (http://www.aap.org), the American Academy of Family Physicians (http://www.aafp.org), and the American College of Obstetricians and Gynecologists (http://www.acog.org).

Footnotes for Figure 20.3, Recommended Immunization Schedule for Persons Aged 0 Through 18 Years—United States, 2015

For further guidance on the use of the vaccines mentioned below, see: http://www.cdc.gov/vaccines/hcp/acip-recs/index.html. For vaccine recommendations for persons 19 years of age and older, see the Adult Immunization Schedule.

Additional information

- For contraindications and precautions to use of a vaccine and for additional information regarding that vaccine, vaccination providers should consult the relevant ACIP statement available online at http://www.cdc.gov/vaccines/hcp/acip-recs/index.html.
- For purposes of calculating intervals between doses, 4 weeks = 28 days. Intervals of 4 months or greater are determined by calendar months.
- Vaccine doses administered 4 days or less before the minimum interval are considered valid. Doses of any vaccine administered ≥5 days earlier than the minimum interval or minimum age should not be counted as valid doses and should be repeated as age-appropriate. The repeat dose should be spaced after the invalid dose by the recommended minimum interval. For further details, see *MMWR, General Recommendations on Immunization and Reports* / Vol. 60 / No. 2; Table 1. Recommended and minimum ages and intervals between vaccine doses, available online at http://www.cdc.gov/mmwr/pdf/rr/rr6002.pdf.
- Information on travel vaccine requirements and recommendations is available at http://wwwnc.cdc.gov/travel/destinations/list.
- For vaccination of persons with primary and secondary immunodeficiencies, see Table 13, "Vaccination of persons with primary and secondary immunodeficiencies," in General Recommendations on Immunization (ACIP), available at http://www.cdc.gov/mmwr/pdf/rr/rr6002.pdf.; and American Academy of Pediatrics. "Immunization in Special Clinical Circumstances," in Pickering LK, Baker CJ, Kimberlin DW, Long SS eds. Red Book: 2012 report of the Committee on Infectious Diseases. 29th ed. Elk Grove Village, IL: American Academy of Pediatrics.

1. **Hepatitis B (HepB) vaccine. (Minimum age: birth)**

Routine vaccination:

At birth:

- Administer monovalent HepB vaccine to all newborns before hospital discharge.
- For infants born to hepatitis B surface antigen (HBsAg)-positive mothers, administer HepB vaccine and 0.5 mL of hepatitis B immune globulin (HBIG) within 12 hours of birth. These infants should be tested for HBsAg and antibody to HBsAg (anti-HBs) 1 to 2 months after completion of the HepB series at age 9 through 18 months (preferably at the next well-child visit).
- If mother's HBsAg status is unknown, within 12 hours of birth administer HepB vaccine regardless of birth weight. For infants weighing less than 2,000 grams, administer HBIG in addition to HepB vaccine within 12 hours of birth. Determine mother's HBsAg status as soon as possible and, if mother is HBsAg-positive, also administer HBIG for infants weighing 2,000 grams or more as soon as possible, but no later than age 7 days.

Doses following the birth dose:

- The second dose should be administered at age 1 or 2 months. Monovalent HepB vaccine should be used for doses administered before age 6 weeks.

continued on page 240

Footnotes for Figure 20.3, *continued from page 239*

- Infants who did not receive a birth dose should receive 3 doses of a HepB-containing vaccine on a schedule of 0, 1 to 2 months, and 6 months starting as soon as feasible. See catch-up schedule.
- Administer the second dose 1 to 2 months after the first dose (minimum interval of 4 weeks), administer the third dose at least 8 weeks after the second dose AND at least 16 weeks after the first dose. The final (third or fourth) dose in the HepB vaccine series should be administered no earlier than age 24 weeks.
- Administration of a total of 4 doses of HepB vaccine is permitted when a combination vaccine containing HepB is administered after the birth dose.

Catch-up vaccination:

- Unvaccinated persons should complete a 3-dose series.
- A 2-dose series (doses separated by at least 4 months) of adult formulation Recombivax HB is licensed for use in children aged 11 through 15 years.
- For other catch-up guidance, see catch-up schedule.

2. **Rotavirus (RV) vaccines. (Minimum age: 6 weeks for both RV1 [Rotarix] and RV5 [RotaTeq])**

Routine vaccination:

Administer a series of RV vaccine to all infants as follows:

1. If Rotarix is used, administer a 2-dose series at 2 and 4 months of age.
2. If RotaTeq is used, administer a 3-dose series at ages 2, 4, and 6 months.
3. If any dose in the series was RotaTeq or vaccine product is unknown for any dose in the series, a total of 3 doses of RV vaccine should be administered.

Catch-up vaccination:

- The maximum age for the first dose in the series is 14 weeks, 6 days; vaccination should not be initiated for infants aged 15 weeks, 0 days or older.
- The maximum age for the final dose in the series is 8 months, 0 days.
- For other catch-up guidance, see catch-up schedule.

3. **Diphtheria and tetanus toxoids and acellular pertussis (DTaP) vaccine. (Minimum age: 6 weeks. Exception: DTaP-IPV [Kinrix]: 4 years)**

Routine vaccination:

- Administer a 5-dose series of DTaP vaccine at ages 2, 4, 6, 15 through 18 months, and 4 through 6 years. The fourth dose may be administered as early as age 12 months, provided at least 6 months have elapsed since the third dose. However, the fourth dose of DTaP need not be repeated if it was administered at least 4 months after the third dose of DTaP.

Catch-up vaccination:

- The fifth dose of DTaP vaccine is not necessary if the fourth dose was administered at age 4 years or older.
- For other catch-up guidance, see catch-up schedule.

4. **Tetanus and diphtheria toxoids and acellular pertussis (Tdap) vaccine. (Minimum age: 10 years for both Boostrix and Adacel)**

Routine vaccination:

- Administer 1 dose of Tdap vaccine to all adolescents aged 11 through 12 years.
- Tdap may be administered regardless of the interval since the last tetanus and diphtheria toxoid-containing vaccine.
- Administer 1 dose of Tdap vaccine to pregnant adolescents during each pregnancy (preferred during 27 through 36 weeks' gestation) regardless of time since prior Td or Tdap vaccination.

Catch-up vaccination:

- Persons aged 7 years and older who are not fully immunized with DTaP vaccine should receive Tdap vaccine as 1 dose (preferably the first) in the catch-up series; if additional doses are needed, use Td vaccine. For children 7 through 10 years who receive a dose of Tdap as part of the catch-up series, an adolescent Tdap vaccine dose at age 11 through 12 years should NOT be administered. Td should be administered instead 10 years after the Tdap dose.
- Persons aged 11 through 18 years who have not received Tdap vaccine should receive a dose followed by tetanus and diphtheria toxoid (Td) booster doses every 10 years thereafter.
- Inadvertent doses of DTaP vaccine:
  - — If administered inadvertently to a child aged 7 through 10 years may count as part of the catch-up series. This dose may count as the adolescent Tdap dose, or the child can later receive a Tdap booster dose at age 11 through 12 years.
  - — If administered inadvertently to an adolescent aged 11 through 18 years, the dose should be counted as the adolescent Tdap booster.
- For other catch-up guidance, see catch-up schedule.

5. ***Haemophilus influenzae*** **type b (Hib) conjugate vaccine. (Minimum age: 6 weeks for PRP-T [ACTHIB, DTaP-IPV/Hib (Pentacel) and Hib-MenCY (MenHibrix)], PRP-OMP [PedvaxHIB or COMVAX], 12 months for PRP-T [Hiberix])**

Routine vaccination:

- Administer a 2- or 3-dose Hib vaccine primary series and a booster dose (dose 3 or 4 depending on vaccine used in primary series) at age 12 through 15 months to complete a full Hib vaccine series.
- The primary series with ActHIB, MenHibrix, or Pentacel consists of 3 doses and should be administered at 2, 4, and 6 months of age. The primary series with PedvaxHib or COMVAX consists of 2 doses and should be administered at 2 and 4 months of age; a dose at age 6 months is not indicated.
- One booster dose (dose 3 or 4 depending on vaccine used in primary series) of any Hib vaccine should be administered at age 12 through 15 months. An exception is Hiberix vaccine. Hiberix should only be used for the booster (final) dose in children aged 12 months through 4 years who have received at least 1 prior dose of Hib-containing vaccine.
- For recommendations on the use of MenHibrix in patients at increased risk for meningococcal disease, please refer to the meningococcal vaccine footnotes and also to *MMWR* February 28, 2014 / 63(RR01);1-13, available at http://www.cdc.gov/mmwr/PDF/rr/rr6301.pdf.

continued on page 242

Footnotes for Figure 20.3, *continued from page 241*

Catch-up vaccination:

- If dose 1 was administered at ages 12 through 14 months, administer a second (final) dose at least 8 weeks after dose 1, regardless of Hib vaccine used in the primary series.
- If both doses were PRP-OMP (PedvaxHIB or COMVAX), and were administered before the first birthday, the third (and final) dose should be administered at age 12 through 59 months and at least 8 weeks after the second dose.
- If the first dose was administered at age 7 through 11 months, administer the second dose at least 4 weeks later and a third (and final) dose at age 12 through 15 months or 8 weeks after second dose, whichever is later.
- If first dose is administered before the first birthday and second dose administered at younger than 15 months, a third (and final) dose should be given 8 weeks later.
- For unvaccinated children aged 15 months or older, administer only 1 dose.
- For other catch-up guidance, see catch-up schedule. For catch-up guidance related to MenHibrix, please see the meningococcal vaccine footnotes and also *MMWR* February 28, 2014 / 63(RR01);1-13, available at http://www.cdc.gov/mmwr/PDF/rr/rr6301.pdf.

Vaccination of persons with high-risk conditions:

- Children aged 12 through 59 months who are at increased risk for Hib disease, including chemotherapy recipients and those with anatomic or functional asplenia (including sickle cell disease), human immunodeficiency virus (HIV) infection, immunoglobulin deficiency, or early component complement deficiency, who have received either no doses or only 1 dose of Hib vaccine before 12 months of age, should receive 2 additional doses of Hib vaccine 8 weeks apart; children who received 2 or more doses of Hib vaccine before 12 months of age should receive 1 additional dose.
- For patients younger than 5 years of age undergoing chemotherapy or radiation treatment who received a Hib vaccine dose(s) within 14 days of starting therapy or during therapy, repeat the dose(s) at least 3 months following therapy completion.
- Recipients of hematopoietic stem cell transplant (HSCT) should be revaccinated with a 3-dose regimen of Hib vaccine starting 6 to 12 months after successful transplant, regardless of vaccination history; doses should be administered at least 4 weeks apart.
- A single dose of any Hib-containing vaccine should be administered to unimmunized* children and adolescents 15 months of age and older undergoing an elective splenectomy; if possible, vaccine should be administered at least 14 days before procedure.
- Hib vaccine is not routinely recommended for patients 5 years or older. However, 1 dose of Hib vaccine should be administered to unimmunized* persons aged 5 years or older who have anatomic or functional asplenia (including sickle cell disease) and unvaccinated persons 5 through 18 years of age with human immunodeficiency virus (HIV) infection.

** Patients who have not received a primary series and booster dose or at least 1 dose of Hib vaccine after 14 months of age are considered unimmunized.*

6. **Pneumococcal vaccines. (Minimum age: 6 weeks for PCV13, 2 years for PPSV23)**

Routine vaccination with PCV13:

- Administer a 4-dose series of PCV13 vaccine at ages 2, 4, and 6 months and at age 12 through 15 months.

- For children aged 14 through 59 months who have received an age-appropriate series of 7-valent PCV (PCV7), administer a single supplemental dose of 13-valent PCV (PCV13).

Catch-up vaccination with PCV13:

- Administer 1 dose of PCV13 to all healthy children aged 24 through 59 months who are not completely vaccinated for their age.
- For other catch-up guidance, see catch-up schedule.

Vaccination of persons with high-risk conditions with PCV13 and PPSV23:

- All recommended PCV13 doses should be administered prior to PPSV23 vaccination if possible.
- For children 2 through 5 years of age with any of the following conditions: chronic heart disease (particularly cyanotic congenital heart disease and cardiac failure); chronic lung disease (including asthma if treated with high-dose oral corticosteroid therapy); diabetes mellitus; cerebrospinal fluid leak; cochlear implant; sickle cell disease and other hemoglobinopathies; anatomic or functional asplenia; HIV infection; chronic renal failure; nephrotic syndrome; diseases associated with treatment with immunosuppressive drugs or radiation therapy, including malignant neoplasms, leukemias, lymphomas, and Hodgkin's disease; solid organ transplantation; or congenital immunodeficiency:
  1. Administer 1 dose of PCV13 if any incomplete schedule of 3 doses of PCV (PCV7 and/or PCV13) were received previously.
  2. Administer 2 doses of PCV13 at least 8 weeks apart if unvaccinated or any incomplete schedule of fewer than 3 doses of PCV (PCV7 and/or PCV13) were received previously.
  3. Administer 1 supplemental dose of PCV13 if 4 doses of PCV7 or other age-appropriate complete PCV7 series was received previously.
  4. The minimum interval between doses of PCV (PCV7 or PCV13) is 8 weeks.
  5. For children with no history of PPSV23 vaccination, administer PPSV23 at least 8 weeks after the most recent dose of PCV13.
- For children aged 6 through 18 years who have cerebrospinal fluid leak; cochlear implant; sickle cell disease and other hemoglobinopathies; anatomic or functional asplenia; congenital or acquired immunodeficiencies; HIV infection; chronic renal failure; nephrotic syndrome; diseases associated with treatment with immunosuppressive drugs or radiation therapy, including malignant neoplasms, leukemias, lymphomas, and Hodgkin's disease; generalized malignancy; solid organ transplantation; or multiple myeloma:
  1. If neither PCV13 nor PPSV23 has been received previously, administer 1 dose of PCV13 now and 1 dose of PPSV23 at least 8 weeks later.
  2. If PCV13 has been received previously but PPSV23 has not, administer 1 dose of PPSV23 at least 8 weeks after the most recent dose of PCV13.
  3. If PPSV23 has been received but PCV13 has not, administer 1 dose of PCV13 at least 8 weeks after the most recent dose of PPSV23.
- For children aged 6 through 18 years with chronic heart disease (particularly cyanotic congenital heart disease and cardiac failure), chronic lung disease (including asthma if treated with high-dose oral corticosteroid therapy), diabetes mellitus, alcoholism, or chronic liver disease, who have not received PPSV23, administer 1 dose of PPSV23. If PCV13 has been received previously, then PPSV23 should be administered at least 8 weeks after any prior PCV13 dose.
- A single revaccination with PPSV23 should be administered 5 years after the first dose to children with sickle cell disease or other hemoglobinopathies; anatomic or functional asplenia; congenital or acquired immunodeficiencies; HIV infection; chronic renal failure; nephrotic syndrome; diseases associated with treatment with

continued on page 244

Footnotes for Figure 20.3, *continued from page 243*

immunosuppressive drugs or radiation therapy, including malignant neoplasms, leukemias, lymphomas, and Hodgkin's disease; generalized malignancy; solid organ transplantation; or multiple myeloma.

7. **Inactivated poliovirus vaccine (IPV). (Minimum age: 6 weeks)**

Routine vaccination:

- Administer a 4-dose series of IPV at ages 2, 4, 6 through 18 months, and 4 through 6 years. The final dose in the series should be administered on or after the fourth birthday and at least 6 months after the previous dose.

Catch-up vaccination:

- In the first 6 months of life, minimum age and minimum intervals are only recommended if the person is at risk of imminent exposure to circulating poliovirus (i.e., travel to a polio-endemic region or during an outbreak).
- If 4 or more doses are administered before age 4 years, an additional dose should be administered at age 4 through 6 years and at least 6 months after the previous dose.
- A fourth dose is not necessary if the third dose was administered at age 4 years or older and at least 6 months after the previous dose.
- If both OPV and IPV were administered as part of a series, a total of 4 doses should be administered,
- Regardless of the child's current age. IPV is not routinely recommended for U.S. residents aged 18 years or older.
- For other catch-up guidance, see catch-up schedule.

8. **Influenza vaccines. (Minimum age: 6 months for inactivated influenza vaccine [IIV], 2 years for live, attenuated influenza vaccine [LAIV])**

Routine vaccination:

- Administer influenza vaccine annually to all children beginning at age 6 months. For most healthy, nonpregnant persons aged 2 through 49 years, either LAIV or IIV may be used. However, LAIV should NOT be administered to some persons, including 1) persons who have experienced severe allergic reactions to LAIV, any of its components, or to a previous dose of any other influenza vaccine; 2) children 2 through 17 years receiving aspirin or aspirin-containing products; 3) persons who are allergic to eggs; 4) pregnant women; 5) immunosuppressed persons; 6) children 2 through 4 years of age with asthma or who had wheezing in the past 12 months; or 7) persons who have taken influenza antiviral medications in the previous 48 hours. For all other contraindications and precautions to use of LAIV, see *MMWR* August 15, 2014 / 63(32);691-697 [40 pages] available at http://www.cdc.gov/mmwr/pdf/wk/mm6332.pdf.

For children aged 6 months through 8 years:

- For the 2014-15 season, administer 2 doses (separated by at least 4 weeks) to children who are receiving influenza vaccine for the first time. Some children in this age group who have been vaccinated previously will also need 2 doses. For additional guidance, follow dosing guidelines in the 2014-15 ACIP influenza vaccine recommendations, *MMWR* August 15, 2014 / 63(32);691–697 [40 pages] available at http://www.cdc.gov/mmwr/pdf/wk/mm6332.pdf.
- For the 2015–16 season, follow dosing guidelines in the 2015 ACIP influenza vaccine recommendations.

For persons aged 9 years and older:

- Administer 1 dose.

9. **Measles, mumps, and rubella (MMR) vaccine. (Minimum age: 12 months for routine vaccination)**

Routine vaccination:

- Administer a 2-dose series of MMR vaccine at ages 12 through 15 months and 4 through 6 years. The second dose may be administered before age 4 years, provided at least 4 weeks have elapsed since the first dose.
- Administer 1 dose of MMR vaccine to infants aged 6 through 11 months before departure from the United States for international travel. These children should be revaccinated with 2 doses of MMR vaccine, the first at age 12 through 15 months (12 months if the child remains in an area where disease risk is high), and the second dose at least 4 weeks later.
- Administer 2 doses of MMR vaccine to children aged 12 months and older before departure from the United States for international travel. The first dose should be administered on or after age 12 months and the second dose at least 4 weeks later.

Catch-up vaccination:

- Ensure that all school-aged children and adolescents have had 2 doses of MMR vaccine; the minimum interval between the 2 doses is 4 weeks.

10. **Varicella (VAR) vaccine. (Minimum age: 12 months)**

Routine vaccination:

- Administer a 2-dose series of VAR vaccine at ages 12 through 15 months and 4 through 6 years. The second dose may be administered before age 4 years, provided at least 3 months have elapsed since the first dose. If the second dose was administered at least 4 weeks after the first dose, it can be accepted as valid.

Catch-up vaccination:

- Ensure that all persons aged 7 through 18 years without evidence of immunity (see *MMWR* 2007 / 56 [No. RR-4], available at http://www.cdc.gov/mmwr/pdf/rr/rr5604.pdf) have 2 doses of varicella vaccine. For children aged 7 through 12 years, the recommended minimum interval between doses is 3 months (if the second dose was administered at least 4 weeks after the first dose, it can be accepted as valid); for persons aged 13 years and older, the minimum interval between doses is 4 weeks.

11. **Hepatitis A (HepA) vaccine. (Minimum age: 12 months)**

Routine vaccination:

- Initiate the 2-dose HepA vaccine series at 12 through 23 months; separate the 2 doses by 6 to 18 months.
- Children who have received 1 dose of HepA vaccine before age 24 months should receive a second dose 6 to 18 months after the first dose.
- For any person aged 2 years and older who has not already received the HepA vaccine series, 2 doses of HepA vaccine separated by 6 to 18 months may be administered if immunity against hepatitis A virus infection is desired.

Catch-up vaccination:

- The minimum interval between the two doses is 6 months.

continued on page 246

Footnotes for Figure 20.3, *continued from page 245*

Special populations:

- Administer 2 doses of HepA vaccine at least 6 months apart to previously unvaccinated persons who live in areas where vaccination programs target older children, or who are at increased risk for infection. This includes persons traveling to or working in countries that have high or intermediate endemicity of infection; men having sex with men; users of injection and non-injection illicit drugs; persons who work with HAV-infected primates or with HAV in a research laboratory; persons with clotting-factor disorders; persons with chronic liver disease; and persons who anticipate close personal contact (e.g., household or regular babysitting) with an international adoptee during the first 60 days after arrival in the United States from a country with high or intermediate endemicity. The first dose should be administered as soon as the adoption is planned, ideally 2 or more weeks before the arrival of the adoptee.

12. **Human papillomavirus (HPV) vaccines. (Minimum age: 9 years for HPV2 [Cervarix] and HPV4 [Gardasil])**

Routine vaccination:

- Administer a 3-dose series of HPV vaccine on a schedule of 0, 1-2, and 6 months to all adolescents aged 11 through 12 years. Either HPV4 or HPV2 may be used for females, and only HPV4 may be used for males.
- The vaccine series may be started at age 9 years.
- Administer the second dose 1 to 2 months after the first dose (minimum interval of 4 weeks); administer the third dose 24 weeks after the first dose and 16 weeks after the second dose (minimum interval of 12 weeks).

Catch-up vaccination:

- Administer the vaccine series to females (either HPV2 or HPV4) and males (HPV4) at age 13 through 18 years if not previously vaccinated.
- Use recommended routine dosing intervals (see Routine vaccination above) for vaccine series catch-up.

13. **Meningococcal conjugate vaccines. (Minimum age: 6 weeks for Hib-MenCY [MenHibrix], 9 months for MenACWY-D [Menactra], 2 months for MenACWY-CRM [Menveo])**

Routine vaccination:

- Administer a single dose of Menactra or Menveo vaccine at age 11 through 12 years, with a booster dose at age 16 years.
- Adolescents aged 11 through 18 years with human immunodeficiency virus (HIV) infection should receive a 2-dose primary series of Menactra or Menveo with at least 8 weeks between doses.
- For children aged 2 months through 18 years with high-risk conditions, see below.

Catch-up vaccination:

- Administer Menactra or Menveo vaccine at age 13 through 18 years if not previously vaccinated.
- If the first dose is administered at age 13 through 15 years, a booster dose should be administered at age 16 through 18 years with a minimum interval of at least 8 weeks between doses.
- If the first dose is administered at age 16 years or older, a booster dose is not needed.

- For other catch-up guidance, see catch-up schedule.

Vaccination of persons with high-risk conditions and other persons at increased risk of disease:

- Children with anatomic or functional asplenia (including sickle cell disease):
  1. Menveo
     - *Children who initiate vaccination at 8 weeks through 6 months:* Administer doses at 2, 4, 6, and 12 months of age.
     - *Unvaccinated children 7 through 23 months:* Administer 2 doses, with the second dose at least 12 weeks after the first dose AND after the first birthday.
     - *Children 24 months and older who have not received a complete series:* Administer 2 primary doses at least 8 weeks apart.
  2. MenHibrix
     - *Children 6 weeks through 18 months:* Administer doses at 2, 4, 6, and 12 through 15 months of age.
     - If the first dose of MenHibrix is given at or after 12 months of age, a total of 2 doses should be given at least 8 weeks apart to ensure protection against serogroups C and Y meningococcal disease.
  3. Menactra
     - *Children 24 months and older who have not received a complete series:* Administer 2 primary doses at least 8 weeks apart. If Menactra is administered to a child with asplenia (including sickle cell disease), do not administer Menactra until 2 years of age and at least 4 weeks after the completion of all PCV13 doses.
- Children with persistent complement component deficiency:
  1. Menveo
     - *Children who initiate vaccination at 8 weeks through 6 months:* Administer doses at 2, 4, 6, and 12 months of age.
     - *Unvaccinated children 7 through 23 months:* Administer 2 doses, with the second dose at least 12 weeks after the first dose AND after the first birthday.
     - *Children 24 months and older who have not received a complete series:* Administer 2 primary doses at least 8 weeks apart.
  2. MenHibrix
     - *Children 6 weeks through 18 months:* Administer doses at 2, 4, 6, and 12 through 15 months of age.
     - If the first dose of MenHibrix is given at or after 12 months of age, a total of 2 doses should be given at least 8 weeks apart to ensure protection against serogroups C and Y meningococcal disease.
  3. Menactra
     - *Children 9 through 23 months:* Administer 2 primary doses at least 12 weeks apart.
     - *Children 24 months and older who have not received a complete series:* Administer 2 primary doses at least 8 weeks apart.
- For children who travel to or reside in countries in which meningococcal disease is hyperendemic or epidemic, including countries in the African meningitis belt or the Hajj, administer an age-appropriate formulation and series of Menactra or Menveo for protection against serogroups A and W meningococcal disease. Prior receipt of MenHibrix is not sufficient for children traveling to the meningitis belt or the Hajj because it does not contain serogroups A or W.

continued on page 248

Footnotes for Figure 20.3, *continued from page 247*

- For children at risk during a community outbreak attributable to a vaccine serogroup, administer or complete an age- and formulation-appropriate series of MenHibrix, Menactra, or Menveo.
- For booster doses among persons with high-risk conditions, refer to *MMWR* 2013 / 62(RR02);1-22, available at http://www.cdc.gov/mmwr/preview/mmwrhtml/rr6202a1.htm.

For other catch-up recommendations for these persons, and complete information on use of meningococcal vaccines, including guidance related to vaccination of persons at increased risk of infection, see *MMWR* March 22, 2013 / 62(RR02);1-22, available at http://www.cdc.gov/mmwr/pdf/rr/rr6202.pdf.

Index

D

E

F

G

H

J

K

L

M

N

O

P

Q

R

W

Y

Z